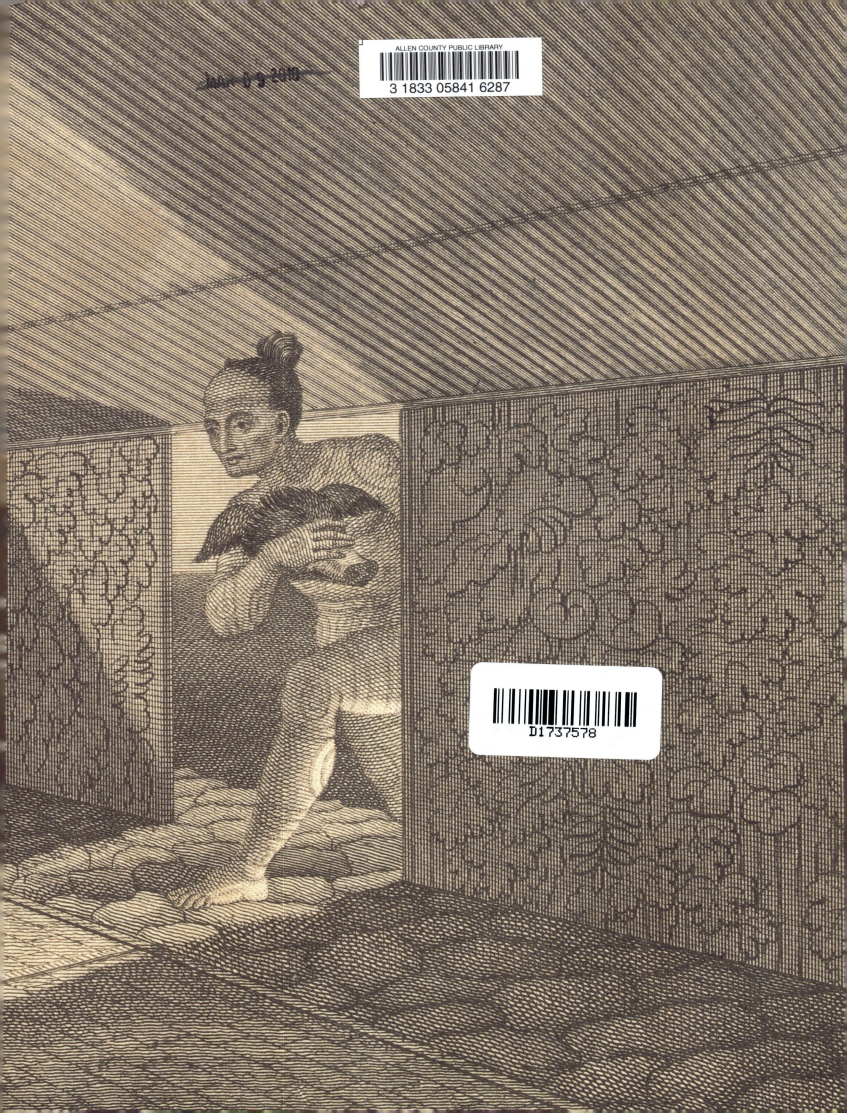

Tattoos
From Paradise
Traditional Polynesian Patterns

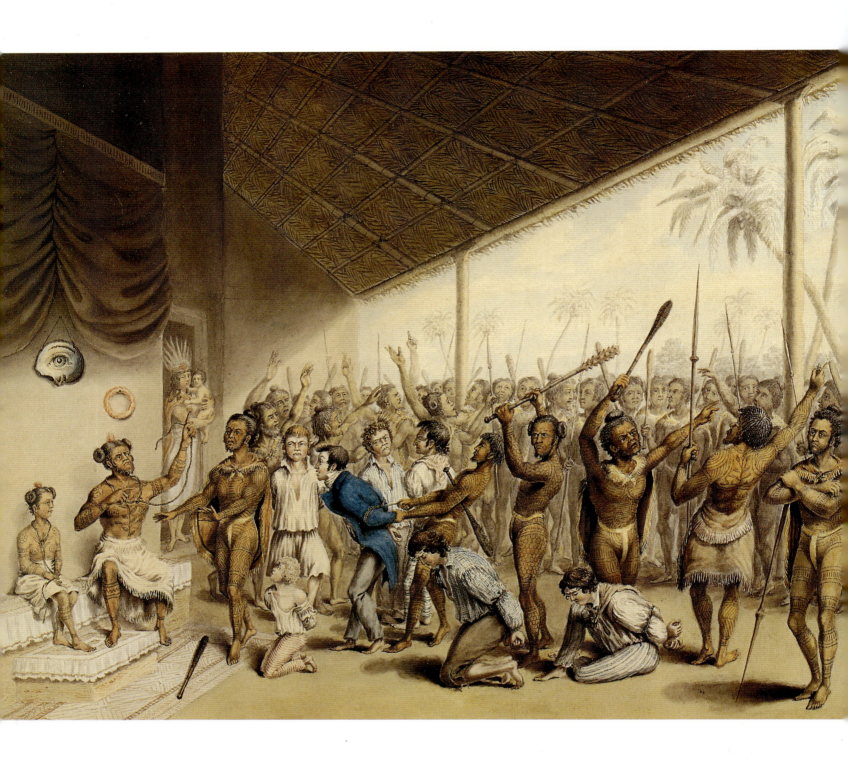

Tattoos From Paradise

Traditional Polynesian Patterns

Mark Blackburn

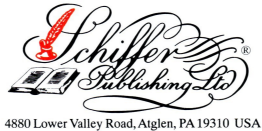

4880 Lower Valley Road, Atglen, PA 19310 USA

Dedication

This book is dedicated to my son Kuhane, whose Tahitian ancestors wore these magnificent *tatau* with pride and honor.

Acknowledgments

I would like to thank the following people for their help along the way: Dr. Terence Barrow whose friendship, knowledge and enthusiasm has helped inspire me to build one of the world's great collections; Dr. David Simmons whose help has always been very much appreciated; Dr. Georgia Lee whose kindness and understanding has been magnificent; Dr. Adrienne Kaeppler whose friendship, knowledge and enthusiasm has enhanced my family's Polynesian experience; Sandy Rosin for her help and enthusiasm in the very beginning; Tricia Allen for her passionate love of the art form; Bernard Nogues for his friendship and help in translation; Ann Johnson for her artwork; Kelly Glouner for her editing skills; my wife Carolyn for putting up with me and my obsessions for the last twenty years; Peter and Nancy Schiffer for believing in the project; Doug Congdon-Martin for his photography; and, lastly, the Polynesian tattoo artists of old.

Artwork photographed for this book is from the collection of Mark and Carolyn Blackburn unless otherwise credited.

Library of Congress Cataloging-in-Publication Data

Blackburn, Mark (Mark A.)
    Tattoos from paradise : traditional Polynesian patterns / Mark Blackburn.
       p. cm.
    Includes bibliographical references.
    ISBN 0-7643-0941-2
    1. Tattooing--Polynesia. 2. Polynesia--social life and customs.
I. Title.
GT2346.P75B57   1999
391.6'5'0996--dc21   99-37553
                                                       CIP

Copyright © 1999 by Mark Blackburn

All rights reserved. No part of this work may be reproduced or used in any form or by any means—graphic, electronic, or mechanical, including photocopying or information storage and retrieval systems—without written permission from the copyright holder.
"Schiffer," "Schiffer Publishing Ltd. & Design," and the "Design of pen and inkwell" are registered trademarks of Schiffer Publishing Ltd.

Designed by Anne Davidsen
Type set in Lydian /Korinna

ISBN: 0-7643-0941-2
Printed in China

Frontispiece: Original watercolor by the English artist George Bray. In this very unusual and disturbing picture, Europeans appear to be led to their execution by various islanders. Illustrated with a cross section of tattoo motifs, ornaments and war clubs all of Polynesian origin, the exact meaning of this picture remains unknown. Signed and dated 1817.

Published by Schiffer Publishing Ltd.
4880 Lower Valley Road
Atglen, PA 19310
Phone: (610) 593-1777; Fax: (610) 593-2002
E-mail: Info@schifferbooks.com
Please visit our web site catalog at
www.schifferbooks.com

This book may be purchased from the publisher.
Include $3.95 for shipping. Please try your bookstore first.
We are always looking for people to write books on new and related subjects. If you have an idea for a book please contact us at the above address.
You may write for a free catalog.

In Europe, Schiffer books are distributed by
Bushwood Books
6 Marksbury Avenue
Kew Gardens
Surrey TW9 4JF England
Phone: 44 (0) 20-8392-8585; Fax: 44 (0) 20-8392-9876
E-mail: info@bushwoodbooks.co.uk
Free postage in the UK. Europe: air mail at cost.

Contents

Introduction	7
New Zealand	9
Hawaii	87
Tahiti	109
Marquesas	117
Easter Island	157
Samoa	173
Tonga	193
Appendix	198
Bibliography	200
Index	203

We tap, yes we tap you a little, yes!
Who knows who will come look at the tattoo of this fellow?
A beautiful maiden will come yes,
To look at the tattoo of this fellow, who knows!
Draw your testicles tight!

—Marquesan Tattoo Chant

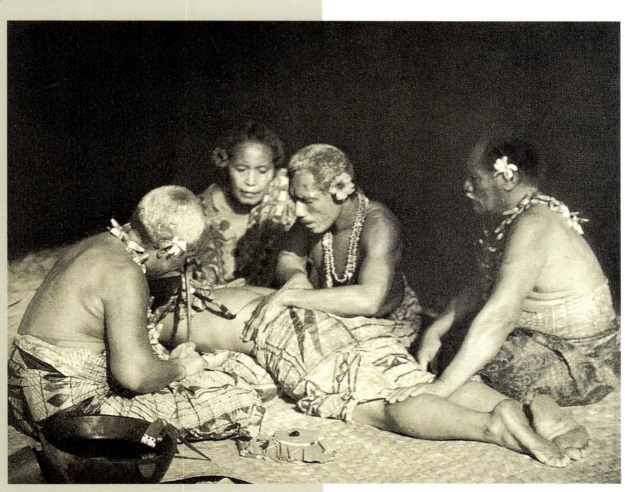

Photograph of a man being tattooed. Photographed by Frances Hubbard Flaherty* in Safune, Savai'i in 1923. This striking image taken during the filming of "Moana of the South Seas: A Romance of the Golden Age" depicts the *tufuga* or tattoo artist at work. Here he is seen starting to tap the first design, known as the *tua* stripe, onto the person's back. His assistants are pulling the skin tight and holding the person down, preventing him from moving. Gelatin silver print on textured paper, probably printed around 1932.

*Frances Hubbard Flaherty (1883-1972) married Robert Flaherty, the arctic explorer, in 1914. With her help he filmed and later released the Eskimo film "Nanook of the North" in 1922. It became such a success that Paramount Pictures asked him to make a film in the location of his choice. He chose Samoa so he could take his family along; they remained there for almost two years filming his masterpiece "Moana of the South Seas: A Romance of the Golden Age." Frances, herself an accomplished photographer, took numerous still photographs that were an integral part of the filmmaking process. She went on to publish several articles on Samoa and to photograph and lecture well after her husband's death in 1951.

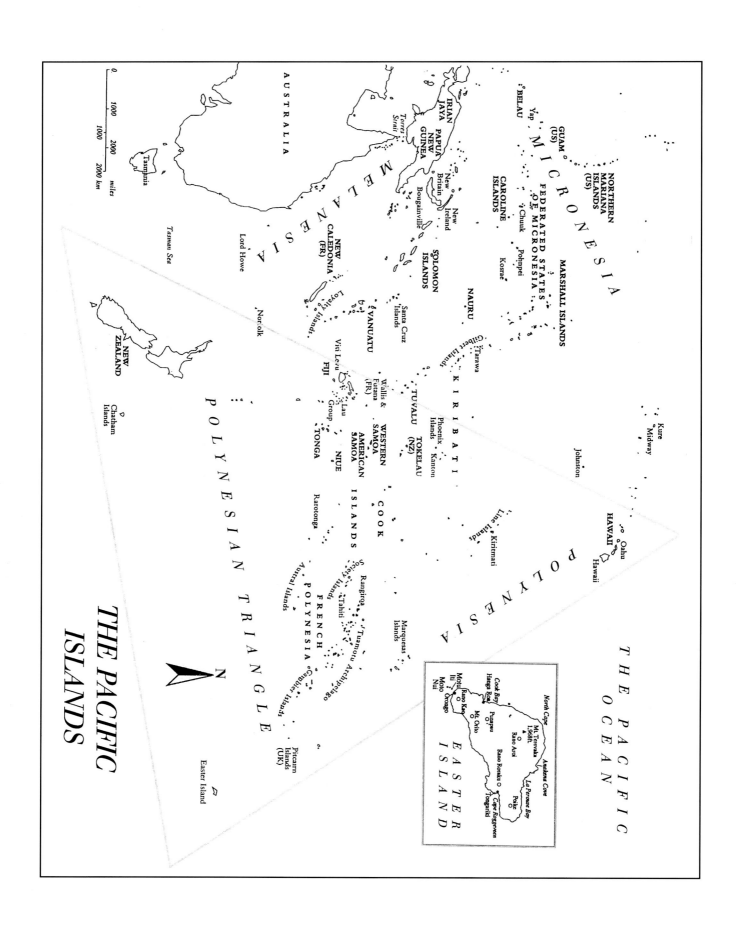

Introduction

TATTOO – The word today stirs up in most of us the fringe element of society, yet there was a place and time when tattoo held the essential spirit and essence of humankind, signifying rank, status, achievement, membership and even events in one's life.

Europeans exploring the vast South Seas in the 18th century encountered the Polynesian Islands for the first time. A highly complex group of cultures existed in this vast area covering one-third of the planet's surface. Within these cultures, tattoo was a highly refined art form as well as an integral strand in the social makeup of things. The word tattoo or *tatau* entered the Western vocabulary for the first time in 1769 when Captain James Cook (1728-1779), on his first voyage of discovery, encountered the native people of Tahiti:[1]

> Both sexes paint their bodys Tattow as it is called in their language, this is done by inlaying colour of black under their skins in such a manner as to be indelible. Some have ill design'd figures of men, birds or dogs, the women generaly have this figure Z simply on every joint of their fingers and toes, the men have it like wise and both have other defferent figures such as circles, crescents & c which they have on their arms and legs. In short they are so various in the application Of these figures that both the quanity and situation of them seem to depend intirely upon the humour of each individual, yet all agree in having their buttocks cover'd with a deep black, over this most have arches drawn one over another as high as their short ribs which are near a quarter of an inch broad; these arches seem to be their great pride as both men and women show them with great pleasure. Their method of Tattowing I shall now describe. The colour they use is lamp black prepared from the smook of a kind of oily nutt used by them instead of candles; the instruments for pricking it under the skin is made of very thin flat pieces of bone or shell, from a quarter of an inch to an inch and a half broad according to the purpose it is to be use'd for and about an inch and a half long, one end is cut into sharp teeth and the other fasten'd to a handle; the teeth are dipped into the black liquor and then drove by quick sharp blows struck upon the handle with a stick for that purpose into the skin so deep that every stroke is followed with a small quanity of blood, the part so marked remains sore for some days before it heals, As this is a painful operation especially the tattowing their buttocks it is perform'd but once in their life time, it is never done until they are 12 or 14 years of age.

Most scholars today believe the tradition of Polynesian tattoo has its origins in the ancient culture of the *Lapita* people who had their beginnings in South Eastern Asia and Melanesia. The initial settlements into the Pacific were achieved by these remarkable and highly skilled voyagers who settled in the island of Tonga and Samoa approximately 1200-200 BC. From these islands the art was spread throughout the rest of Polynesia. What is most remarkable about these *Lapita* people was the use of pottery[2] that vanished shortly after the time of contact, with the exception of neighboring Fiji. The relation that this culture has to tattooing is very significant, as the pieces of pottery produced by these people were decorated with incised design motifs. Being both curvilinear as well as rectilinear in nature, these are most certainly the immediate source of both Austronesian as well as Polynesian tattoo, the patterns consisting of chevrons, spirals, geometric elements, sea creatures, stylized masks, and others.[3]

There are two types of traditional tattooing found in Polynesia: smooth and grooved. Smooth tattooing was practiced in all the islands and was a way of pricking the skin with a toothed comb carrying a pigment leaving a smooth, blemish-free skin. The other, which is the grooved method, was practiced only by the Maori people of New Zealand and consisted of literally carving the skin to make a groove and then inserting the pigment. This type of tattooing became the main fashion of the Maori, replacing the smooth skin type that was occasionally seen on the North Island.

The Polynesians are one of the most resourceful cultures ever to exist on this planet. These Stone Age people evolved into a well-balanced society based upon gardening and fishing. They had skilled artisans and craftsmen, with their ingenious artistic skills being among the finest of all the tribal peoples of the world. Their religious life was based upon a complex set of rituals and ceremonies. The non-visual arts consisted of oratory, genealogical chants, song, dance, poetry and storytelling, with the relating of deeds of the gods and ancestors being incredibly diverse. They had no written script for recording events;[4] priests and learned men were responsible for passing on tribal lore and history.

With the coming of the Europeans, the Polynesians cast aside their traditional culture. In all parts of Polynesia missionaries encouraged their converts to destroy anything that belonged to their pagan past. In this context, it is a miracle that this art of Polynesia has survived. Today, tattoo has taken on a meaning as never before. It has a new role to play in the revival of the Polynesian spirit – promoting the vitality of these cultures into the next millenium. It is with great pleasure and admiration for these remarkable people that I present the reader with the following pages.

Endnotes
[1] The author has taken the liberty of keeping quotes from the 18th century in their original Old English format wherever possible, adding to the feeling of that time period.
[2] *Lapita* pottery shards have also been found in other areas of the Pacific, including the southeast Solomon Islands and New Caledonia.
[3] These patterns are also most certainly the source of design elements in war club decoration, barkcloth and rock art, including the unique barkcloth images from Easter Island.
[4] The only writing or script being the *rongorongo* tablets of Easter Island. The glyphs incised on these tablets appear to be genealogical in nature.

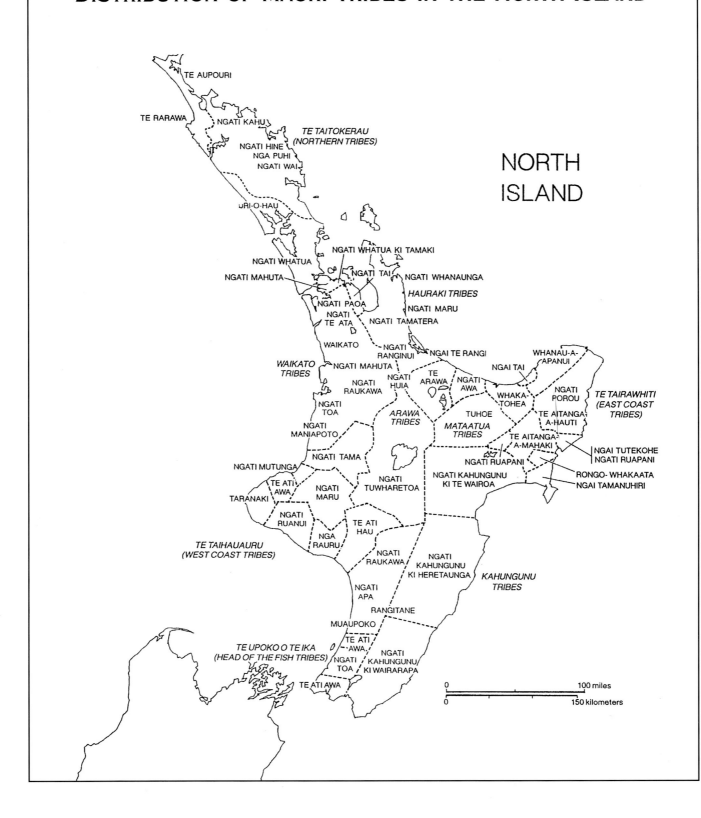

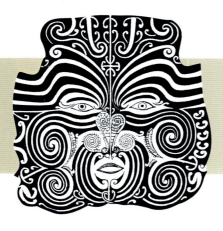

NEW ZEALAND
Aotearoa

Aotearoa, Land of the Long White Cloud, is an isolated group of two islands 1,200 miles southeast of Australia and a similar distance south-southwest of Tonga. The two islands are mountainous, especially the South Island where the Southern Alps rise above the 12,000-foot level at Mt. Cook. The North Island has a vast area of rich lowlands that are more suitable for agriculture, especially for the growing of *kumura* (sweet potato), which was a mainstay in the traditional Maori diet of the 18th and 19th centuries. Due to climatic and topographical features the early Polynesian Maori inhabitants mainly settled in this rich fertile North Island, which is where the majority of the present-day population of Maori and *pakeha*[1] resides.

The first Polynesian inhabitants of New Zealand originally came from Tahiti and later the Marquesas around 1000 AD, although oral traditions conflict with this widely accepted place of origin. In traditional Maori beliefs it is held that a great fleet of canoes arrived from the *Hawaiki* homeland sometime in the 14th century.

The first known European visitor was the Dutch explorer Tasman (1603-1659). He arrived in December 1642 and lost four of his men in a skirmish with the Maori in Murderer's Bay before sailing up the west coast of the North Island and on to Tonga.[2]

There was no further contact until Captain Cook arrived in Poverty Bay in October 1769. His first impression is recorded in his journal as follows:

> We saw in the Bay several Canoes, People upon the shore and some houses in the Country. The land on the Sea-Coast is high with white steep clifts and back inland are very high mountains, the face of the Country is of a hilly surface and appears to be cloathed with wood and Vendure.

He spent six months circumnavigating both islands, preparing remarkably accurate charts and contacting Maori at various points on his journey. His first meeting, though, turned bloody and several Maori were killed.

During this first voyage, Sir Joseph Banks (1743-1820), Captain Cook's naturalist, was one of the first to record the art of Maori tattoo. When he was shown some tattooing tools, he remarked:

> One of the old men here shewd us the instruments with which they stain their bodies which was exactly like those used at Otahite. They had a much larger quanity of Amoco or black stains on their bodies or faces: almost universally they had a broad spiral on each buttock and many had their thighs almost entirely black, small lines only being left untouched so that they looked like stripd breaches.

The Maori people living in this period of contact were one of the most advanced cultures in Polynesia. Drawing from a very rich and bountiful environment they were able to produce a complex material culture rivaling or surpassing many cultures of a similar nature. During this "classic" period unique art styles evolved with elaborate and richly carved ornaments, architecture and weaponry. Even clothing was a highly evolved art form with a wide wardrobe of cloaks, capes, kilts, loin-cloths and belts made from the flax plant and ornamented with dog hair and bird feathers.

Maori society was a stratified affair with numerous tribal groups. Two main classes of people were always present in each tribe, one being the senior *rangatira* class and the other the common class of people or *tutua*. Marriages were usually arranged in this senior class of people, and strict incest rules were enforced to preserve purity of lineage. All tasks in the tribal group were under the guidance of the elders, men being regimented to the tasks of hunting, fishing, building and fighting, while women performed their duties of cooking, food, fuel gathering and weaving, and slaves captured in war performed the more menial duties. In this "classic" period the groups lived in well-constructed villages with storehouses, individual dwellings and chiefs' houses. When threatened by a neighboring tribe, they retired to their defensive fortifications or *pas* for protection. These fortifications were remarkable, with elaborate earthworks that became even more complex with more and more palisades added during European times.[3]

The linked aspects of *mana*[3a] and *tapu* were always present as in all Polynesian cultures. The chief, usually the senior male of the most important family and lineage, was imbued with great *mana* by virtue of the purity of his descent from revered and, in some cases, deified ancestors. This *mana* was an inherited quality that could be increased by his skill in war or the way in which he held the tribal unit together.

Tapu, which was intimately bound with *mana*, was the concept of personal sanctity relating to people of rank. Because of a chief's supposed lineal descent from ancestral deities, he was revered, and the *tapu* system provided a channel for his reverence. The head was considered to be the most *tapu* part of the body and particular care had to be exercised in tattooing and even eating.

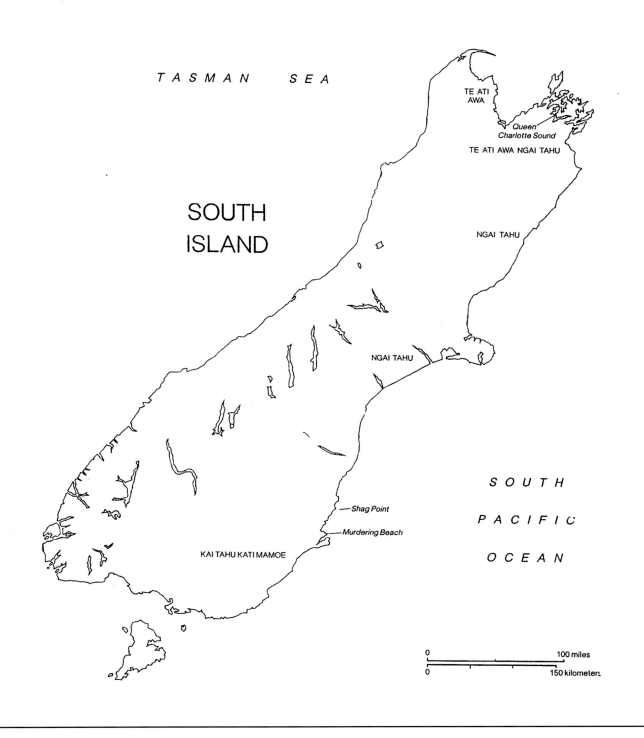

Many activities had *tapu* associations with a strict set of rules that would apply. The infringement of *tapu* brought a state of psychological pollution and physical vulnerability. Many things were explained as a subject of *tapu* violations such as sickness and death. Cleansing rituals with incantations could be used to reverse the *tapu* transgression. Every aspect of daily life was affected by these *tapus*. The only person who could reverse these transgressions was a *tohunga* or, in lay terms, a priest. The *tohunga* was the "expert" who was a repository of tribal lore relating to *tapu*, genealogies, and rituals; he was the link between the earthly and spiritual worlds. Every activity from birth to death had these *tapu* associations, but the Maori did not live in constant fear for there was a multitude of rituals that could be used to rectify *tapu* transgressions. Early Europeans did not understand this concept of *tapu* and unintended violations led to disputes and warfare, giving the Maori people a reputation for unprovoked aggression that was not always deserved.

The Maori pantheon of gods included the major deities recognized in most parts of Polynesia. *Tane,* the forest-life god, was the principal god, probably due to the great dependence of the Maori on the forests and its products. The other gods were *Tu*, god of war and hunting; *Rongo*, god of agriculture and peace; *Tangaroa*, god of sea and fishing; *Tawhirimatea*, god of voyaging and the wind; and *Haumiatiketike*, god of the bracken fern.

With the arrival of Europeans, who came in the form of whalers, traders, sealers, settlers and the like, the Maori were thrust into turmoil. They made powerful alliances with them, but soon trinkets and clothing were not enough, and a brisk trade in muskets allowed the Nga Puhi under Hingi Hika to raid the whole of the North Island in the 1820s. The increased demand for muskets to redress these raids led to an extensive trade in flax, timber, and even preserved human heads.[4] The arrival of the musket also produced an extreme political imbalance, fragmenting tribes and their land, thus making it easier for the *pakeha* to obtain settlement.

The history of the Maori people during this first half of the 19th century was also greatly changed by the gradual conversion of tribes to Christianity. Numerous mission posts were established, and the Nga Puhi were among the first to convert and spread the gospel of peace, using it as a political tool to pre-empt the reprisal raids of the other tribes who were arming for this purpose.

The treaty signing at Waitangi in February 1840 marked the end of the Maoris' political position when the great majority of Maori chiefs set their marks to paper, which established supreme British colonial sovereignty. However, this was not the final attempt at pacification as this weakening caused numerous episodes of defiance.

Fighting broke out in various areas during the "Maori Wars" period in the 1860s resulting in the Maori succumbing to superior arms and numbers. This indiscriminate seizure of Maori land was pronounced in 1927 at a Royal Commission, and the Maoris' original defense of Waitara[5] hence was justified, but this hardly helped the Maori people

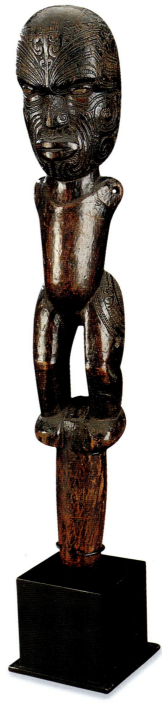

"*Karetao*" or Jumping Jack. Many people consider these to be toys but they are often much more than that. This example, like most known pieces, has lost its movable arms, which would be moved by a cord as a song was sung. Many of them are identified as individuals whose song or songs about them are sung while the operator holds the figure and moves the arms in time to the rhythm. According to noted Maori scholar Dr. D. R. Simmons,* some of these figures are not identified and were more general, but the figure shown here is clearly identified as a *kohere*, a chief placed over a tribal area to lead his people. Further, Dr. Simmons states that the forehead moko design is that of a *kohere* who has authority over the southern area of the tribal lands. This individual's father was of Te Aitanga a Mahaki, his mother of Ngati Porou. The southern area of the tribe is where part of the town of Gisborne now stands. The figure has one tattooed buttock, the sign of a *tohunga* or expert who had protected knowledge. His expertise is shown with the design elements in the moko on the chin. From the Te Aitanga a Mahaki tribe. Wood with paua shell. Height: 21-1/2 inches. Late 18th/early 19th century.
* Personal communication, 1994.

nearly sixty years later. The vast influx of settlers to New Zealand was the root of this problem. It is estimated that the population of settlers grew from 2,000 in 1840 to 600,000 in 1890, while the Maori declined from an estimated 100,000 at the time of Cook's first visit in 1769 to 42,000 in 1890. The Maori population was seen as a "dying race" at the turn of the century, but with the development of the Young Maori Party hope was soon to be seen.

The sense of Maori pride became more evident in *pakeha* society with the advent of a renaissance of Maori arts and crafts and the formation of the School of Art at Rotorua in the 1920s. Notable Maori men during this time period were Sir Peter Buck and Sir Apirana Ngata who brought the plight of their fellow man to the forefront. Today there is much focus on traditional Maori society and how it relates to the *pakeha,* with renewed emphasis on the Maori language. Many Maori land claims are currently before the high courts of New Zealand. Although the main problem for the present-day Maori population may be the high birth rate and burgeoning unemployment, with a stronger-than-ever self-identity, the Maori people will as a race be prepared to face the next century with even greater promise and vigor.

New Zealand Tattooing – *moko*

Traditional Maori tattooing consisted of two basic types: smooth and grooved. The smooth type was fairly rare and found only in the northern Maori; it consisted of pricking the skin with a toothed tattooing comb carrying a dark pigment and is very similar to other Polynesian tattooing. In the latter part of the 19th and 20th centuries, many Maori people being tattooed - especially females - would have the moko applied with the use of darning needles leaving a tattoo that was smooth to the touch.

The grooved type of tattooing was much more prevalent in traditional Maori culture and involved carving the skin. In a manuscript written in Maori sometime before 1853 by Te Rangikaheke of the Ngani Rangiwewehe tribe of Te Arawa, it is described in detail by the following excerpt:[6]

It is the chisel which cuts before the cut there is the drawing, the putting on of the pattern. Drawing is the beginning of tattooing. Afterwards the tohunga takes up the chisel and the mallet. Then it starts, the first chisel struck does not touch the skin. It is a big chisel, a broad chisel. When he arrives at the curves he takes a narrow chisel to use in the curves by the eyes. The first tattooing is an opening of the way, a cutting of the skin, of the flesh to divide it, in order to open a groove. When the way is opened then the tohunga takes the notched chisel. Then the tohunga takes the charcoal and the tow in one hand. The chisel is in this hand, the left. In the right hand is the mallet, the charcoal and the tow, three things in one hand. The notched chisel is to notch the face to make the charcoal hold. This is the second chisel, the opening

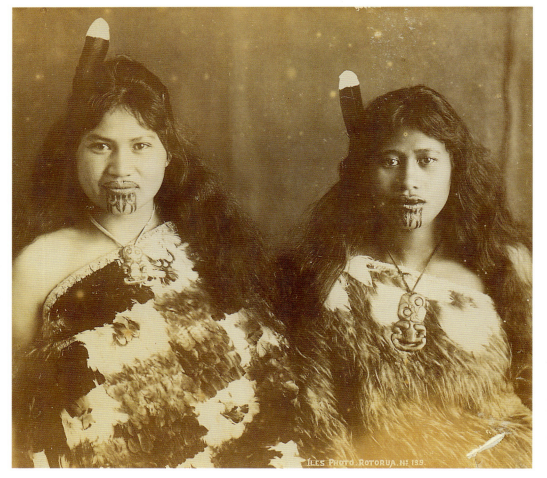

"Unknown Women of Rotorua Area of North Island." A typical photo showing two Arawa ladies with *hei tiki* ornaments and feather cloaks. Original albumen photograph circa 1890s by Iles.

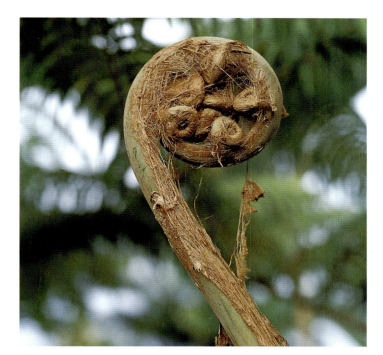

Tree fern. Ferns played a very important part in Maori life, with the bracken root being a staple food as well as being used for building and fencing. The fern could sometimes be a verbal symbol of chieftainship in the Maori language. At least forty-five kinds of spirals are used in Maori carving, the greatest elaboration being found in Auckland, Bay of Plenty and East Coast areas. Like carving, Maori tattoo or *moko* spirals more than likely had their origins in this fern.

is the one which cuts. A broad chisel is used again until the temple is reached, that to the eyes, when a narrow chisel is taken again to do the curves right and is also right for the pakati."[7]

As with all tattooing, it was a very painful process. In the case of a full facial moko for a chief, it would take around a year to complete due to the necessity of allowing one part of the face to heal before operating on another. In an account by Reverend Taylor,[8] he describes a person who was unmercifully tattooed during a war causing his wounds to become so inflamed that the person died a horrific death.

The basic elements of Maori tattoo design were the *koru* and the spiral. The word *koru* is defined in Williams' *Dictionary of the Maori Language* as an adjective meaning "folded, coiled, looped." As a noun the word means "a bulbed motif or scroll painting." There are many schools of thought as to what this design element represents, but the most prevailing is the unfolding of a tree fern frond or curling wave. The spiral, on the other hand, is the most distinctive design element in Maori art. It can be found everywhere and in all time periods in both woodcarving as well as tattoo. As a design element it is closely paralleled in other areas of the nearby world, such as New Guinea and Borneo. Like the *koru*, it had its origin in the tree fern or wave.

The chisels, or *uhi,* used in traditional moko were made from various sources: a seabird wing bone, a shark's tooth, and stone and hardwood that were worked down to fine points. The mallet or *he mahoe* was usually made of whalebone or hardwood. Often the mallet had a broad flattened surface at one end used to wipe away the blood that would interfere with the artist's work. The artist sometimes held in his hand a piece of flax dipped into the pigment that was applied to the incisions. The pigment or *narahu* was made of burnt and powdered resin of the Kauri pine, Kahikatea or Koromico. In early accounts, these resins were often described as charcoal and were said to have produced the finest tint of blue-black color that was so highly esteemed. In some rare cases, a vegetable caterpillar known in the Maori language as *aweto hotete* was used. This, too, was burnt to produce a resin or charcoal that was applied to the incisions. One of the key ingredients in these pigments was oil or dogs' fat, which would help set the dye in place. Gunpowder was also often used as a pigment, especially with the onset of the musket trade in the 1820s.

During the time when a person was being tattooed, he was subject to a strict set of *tapus* in which the initiate was not allowed to speak; eating was not allowed without his attendants who brought him his food as he was not allowed to touch it. It was thought that whoever raised a finger to his mouth during this time period would be invaded by *atuas* or demons and would be eaten alive. The Reverend Taylor describes it as follows:

> During the time of tapu he could not be touched by anyone, nor even put his own hand to his head; but he was fed by another who was appointed for the purpose, or took up his food with his mouth from a small stage with his hands behind him, or by a fernstalk, and thus conveyed it to his mouth. In drinking water, the water was poured in a very expert manner from a calabash into his mouth, or on his hands when he needed it for washing; so that he should not touch the vessel which otherwise could not have been used again for ordinary purposes.

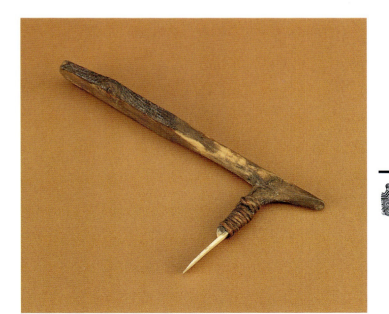

Tattooing tool, "*uhi.*" Bird bone blade bound with flax to wood handle. Early 19th century. Formerly in the Hooper Collection #185. Total length: 4-1/2 inches.

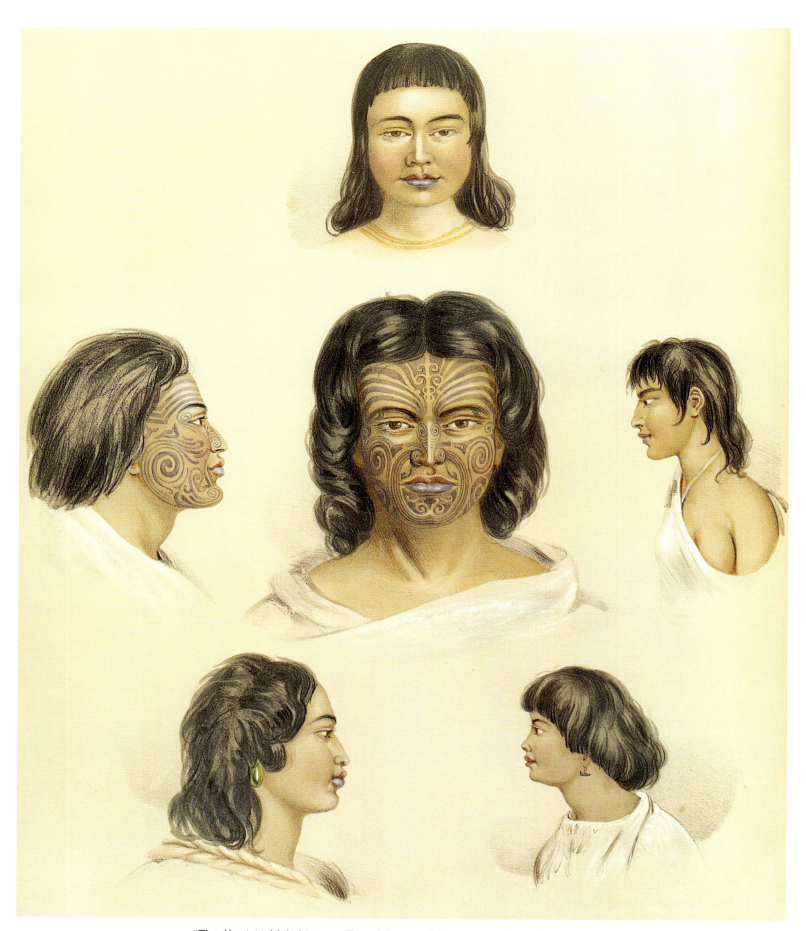

"The Aboriginal Inhabitants – Typical Portraits." Drawn from life by George Angas, 1844. The portraits depicted here show all the design elements in Maori facial tattoo or moko. Shown in the center portrait is the classic *koru*-based design elements. The lips also are tattooed with horizontal lines. In the female portraits, the very simple lower lip tattoo is shown; this was prevalent in some tribal areas at the time. Original lithograph from two-volume set published in 1846 entitled *The New Zealanders Illustrated* by George French Angas.

Sex and washing were to be abstained from for a period of several days after the moko was applied due to the strict nature of the *tapu* system. Many changes were to come along in artistic expression with the advent of the Europeans' introduction of iron. In both wood carving and traditional moko there was an immediate flowering of styles. The iron *uhi* allowed the Maori artist to work at a faster speed with much finer and detailed work being the result. Soon iron replaced all the traditional Maori forms of *uhi* and decadence in Maori art styles began to appear.

Today there are many schools of thought in both the Maori and academic communities on who was tattooed in traditional Maori culture and for what reasons. It is the general opinion, however, that moko was, among other things, a badge of distinction. It is also an identification mark, recording various events in one's life such as exploits in war.

Various styles of moko also signified rank. It is proposed by some academics that distinction of rank can be traced in each moko. It is also said that by interpreting the symbols of the moko it is possible to establish the *mana* and status of its wearer, his lines of descent and tribal affiliations, thus making the moko his or her tribal signature. When the noted Maori chief Te Pehi Kupe visited England in 1826, he made the following remark: "Europee man write with pen his name –Te Pehi's is here."[9] He pointed to his forehead.

Moko styles were in a state of flux especially around the time of the first European contacts. The changes were due to many things, but primarily to inter-tribal contact. This was especially the case in the late 18th century when northern raids were sweeping down the eastern coast to Hauraki. It was at this time that the northern fashion of smooth skin tattoo or *puhoro* was replaced by the grooved *whakairo* tattoo. As this grooved tattoo, which was primarily based upon spiral forms, moved north, the buttock tattoo of this area became the general adornment of warriors of the south.

With the arrival of the first missionaries, male moko came under widespread attack. Numerous early missionary accounts are full of references to this "heathen practice," yet in an odd turn of events it appears the missionaries actually sanctioned a certain type of tattooing. Beginning around 1840, recently baptized converts were tattooed with their baptismal names on their arms. This strange practice was performed by the missionaries to officially mark their converts and acted as a kind of brand. In an account published in 1859 by A.S. Thomson,[10] he describes the following occurrence in the practice of tattooing:

> Tattooing is now going out of fashion, partly from the influence of the missionaries, who describe it as the Devil's art, but chiefly from the example of settlers.

This being said, male moko did have a minor revival during the Maori Wars period of the 1860s, although primarily as a point of defiance against the British and European settlers. By the 1920s the last of the tattooed men of old had died, marking the passing of an era.

With the onset of the decline of male tattooing, female moko was becoming more popular. Prior to this time period, however, various types of women's tattooing were seen; the first recording of a female tattoo was by artist Sydney Parkinson on Captain Cook's voyage in 1769. These first recorded tattoos were quite unusual, one being a neck tattoo, the other being a tattoo of the buttock. Between the years 1820 and 1840, female moko took over as a marker for families of rank. By the 1840s, female moko had reached its height with great variation. In the north, it was just lip tattoo and lines on the chin, lips and forehead or nose, and sometimes legs in the central North Island. It is also recorded that in the Otago area of the South Island women were sometimes tattooed like men, although this was rare.

Female tattooing continued, with various revivals including the first being recorded in 1875. Around the turn of the century a new technique replaced the bone (or later steel) blades used in female tattooing with the use of darning needles. In 1910, another innovation was the use of "grouped" darning needles leaving a heavier pattern in the tattoo. By 1920 there was such a demand for tattooing that some of the practitioners resorted to mass tattooing to satisfy the demand. Some of the more famous practitioners of this time period were Herewini of Ngati Porou, Aterea of Tuhoe, Kuhukuhu of Waikato, Anaru Makiwhara of Ngai Tai and Tame Poata of Ngati Porou.

Traditional female tattooing was recorded as being last practiced in 1953, although that did not stop some men and women from using the services of professional *pakeha* tattoo artists. Today there is a renewed interest in moko with many Maori having it applied by both Maori and *pakeha* practitioners. Moko today is worn as in the past and serves as an expression of these proud people, the people from the land of the long white cloud…

> You may lose your most valuable property through misfortune in various ways…your house, your weaponry, your spouse, and other treasures. You may be robbed of all that you cherish. But of your moko, you cannot be deprived, except by death. It will be your ornament and your companion until your final day.
> Netana Whakaari of Waimana, 1921

Endnotes

[1] Pakeha is a Maori language term for a person of European descent.
[2] In an interesting note, there is no mention in Tasman's journal of the Maori people having been tattooed. Why there is no description baffles the author unless the contact was so brief and so bloody that it was not noticed.
[3] The Maori use of extensive earthworks, etc., was adopted by the West with the advent of World War One, hence the use of trench warfare.
[3a] *Mana*- an Austronesian word used throughout Polynesia to indicate a spiritual power or life force that can be vested in people or objects.
[4] This trade in preserved human heads led to bogus post-mortem tattoo work on the unfortunate slave.
[5] Waitara was one of many tribal lands occupied by the English military, which led to the era known as the "Maori Wars."
[6] This according to the Maori scholar David Simmons in his book *Maori Tattoo* published by the Bush Press, Auckland, New Zealand, 1989.
[7] Maori word translating "As between the line notches."
[8] Reverend Richard Taylor studied the Maori culture at length and in 1855 authored *New Zealand and Its Inhabitants* published in London by Wertheim and Macintosh.
[9] When the treaty of Waitangi was signed in 1840 many of the Maori chiefs inscribed his own moko on the document as his way of recording his signature.
[10] *The Story of New Zealand* published by John Murray, London, 1859.

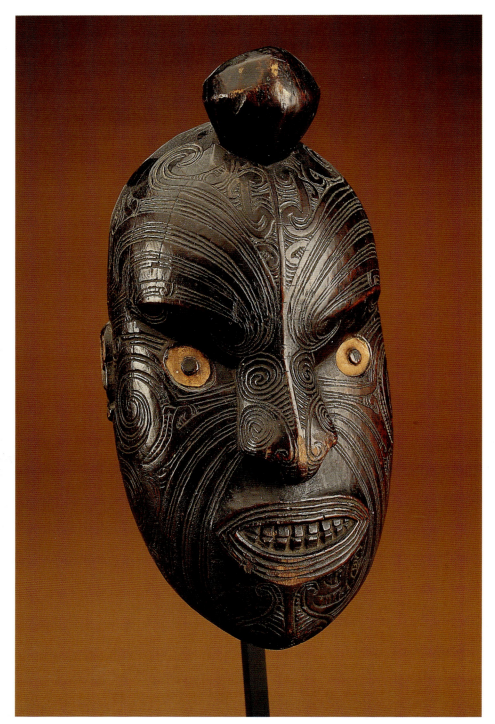

Carved wooden head. This intriguing piece has caused a great deal of speculation as to whether it is a memorial head, the primary purpose being a substitution for lost or damaged preserved human head, or a gable mask (*koruru*) from a house.* Carved heads like this were also used in the decoration of war canoes and were attached to the underside of the bow. Carved with stone tools or soft iron in the late 18th or early 19th century, it is carved in the Hawkes Bay–East Coast style of the North Island. Dr. D. R. Simmons states** that it is his opinion the moko is that of a very high chief and the design on the left (your right) chin is of a person who was a member of the council of high chiefs. He was the Chief, the eldest son of his father, who has succeeded his father but was also given a higher rank because of his achievements. His tribe was Ngati Kahungunu of the particular section known as Pourangahua who combine lines from the original pre-Kahungunu settlers, Kahungunu, the Tuhoe people of Urewera and Tuwharetoa of Taupo. Dr. Simmons further states that it seems that he would belong on the genealogical line of the Taupo and Hawkes Bay Chief Wi Tipuna and was a descendant of Tamarautu, whose descendant *hapu* is named Ngati Tamarautu. Wi Tipuna was living at Papuni, the area occupied by Pourangahua in the Ruakituri valley behind Wairoa on the East Coast, Papuni being the lake. Wi Tipuna was involved in a fierce fight during the "musket wars" around 1820. This invaluable information was given to Dr. Simmons by Te Riria, who is a present-day descendant of Wi Tupuna. The author acquired this piece at auction in London from a small auction house where it had been brought in for valuation and eventual sale by a elderly widow who said it had been hanging in a regimental meeting house for years. How it came to England is anyone's guess, but most likely it was "brought home" by someone involved in the Maori Wars. Wood with paper inlaid eyes. Height: 9-5/8 inches.

*Dr. Simmons has speculated that the head has been removed from a *pou tokomanawa*, a center post of a chief's house and the hollow at the back of the head was used to contain a life force piece such as some dog hair or jade.
**Personal communication, 1992.

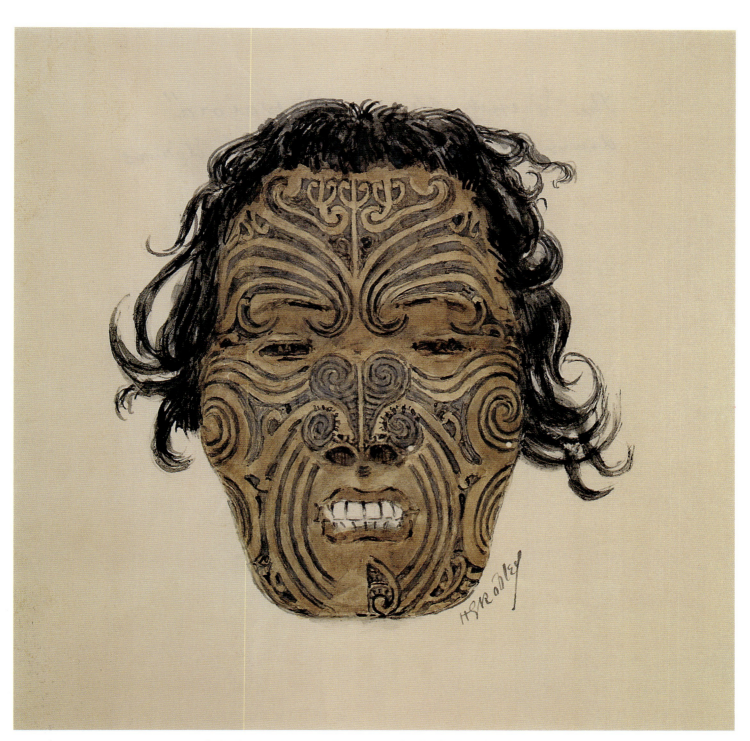

Original watercolor by Major General Horatio Robley.* In this picture a preserved dried head is depicted with an unusual *wairau* or chin design. Robley was quite fascinated with these preserved heads and had over 35 of them in his personal collection. Inscribed on reverse, "The 1/8th inch space waiora down profile divides all patterns." Circa 1900. See page 18 for further information.

*Major General Robley (1840-1930) was a high ranking military man who made a visual record of the wars with the Maori. He is best known, though, for his work on Maori moko and was author of the classic work entitled *Moko* published in 1896. He was an accomplished watercolor artist and illustrated this book with over 180 drawings. In 1915 he published another Book entitled *Pounamu: Notes on New Zealand Greenstone.*

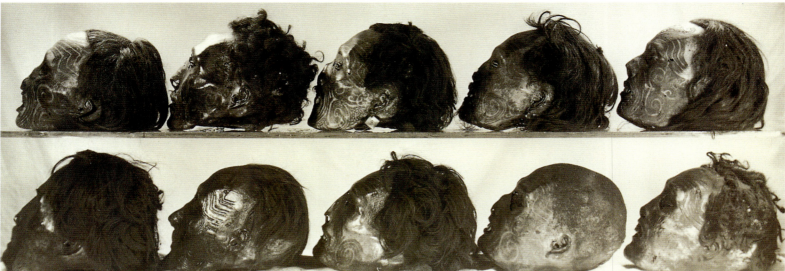

Maori Skulls. From Anthropological Museum, University of Aberdeen. Photographed by Anatomy Dept. 12 June 1946.

Original photograph entitled "Maori Skulls – from Anthropological Museum, University of Aberdeen. Photographed by Anatomy Dept. 12 June 1946." An unusual frontal view showing preserved dried heads with elaborate mokos. Heads of beloved chiefs or other tribesmen of notable rank who died in peacetime or in war were preserved. Given a place of honor, they were treasured as family, tribal or memorial relics. Heads of important foes were also kept by the tribe and were continually abused and suffered the full realm of indignities. To preserve a head, the head would be severed at the neck and the skin would be carefully dissected from the underlying skull. The flesh then would be carefully scraped away. At this point, the skin only would be attached to the skull at the nasal cartilage; it then would be repositioned over the skull. The next and final step involved a lengthy process of smoking interspersed with repeated oilings. In the early part of the 19th century, a brisk European market in preserved heads began. The practice of using heads of enemies as objects of barter - especially for muskets - quickly ensued. According to Hamilton,* all the existing preserved heads were quickly snapped up, leading to a high demand that local Maori chiefs quickly filled. They sought to meet this demand by offering tattooed slaves whose heads would be ready in three days, the price being a casket of powder each. The trade reached its peak in 1831 when Governor Darling of New South Wales Australia imposed a forty pound fine on anyone importing "baked heads" to that province. It is interesting to note that there exists only one female preserved head as indicated by the characteristic chin tattooing. It is also estimated that there are hundreds of these heads in existence, most housed in museum collections.**

*Augustus Hamilton was the author of a book published by the New Zealand Institute in 1896 entitled *The Art Workmanship of the Maori Race in New Zealand*. This book, which is profusely illustrated, was the first in-depth study of traditional Maori Arts and Crafts.

**Because of the sensitivity and respect granted to the Maori people today, most heads have been taken off view at the world's museums. Leaders of the Maori are currently in talks with many institutions where these heads are stored, negotiating their return to the Maori people. The author, although offered preserved heads in the past, likewise has respected the wishes of the Maori people and supports the Maoris' efforts to reclaim their ancestors.

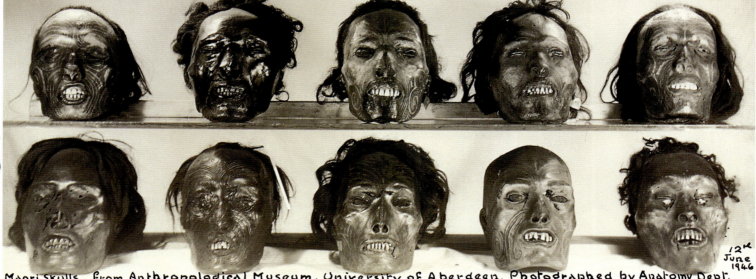

Maori Skulls. From Anthropological Museum. University of Aberdeen. Photographed by Anatomy Dept. 12 June 1946.

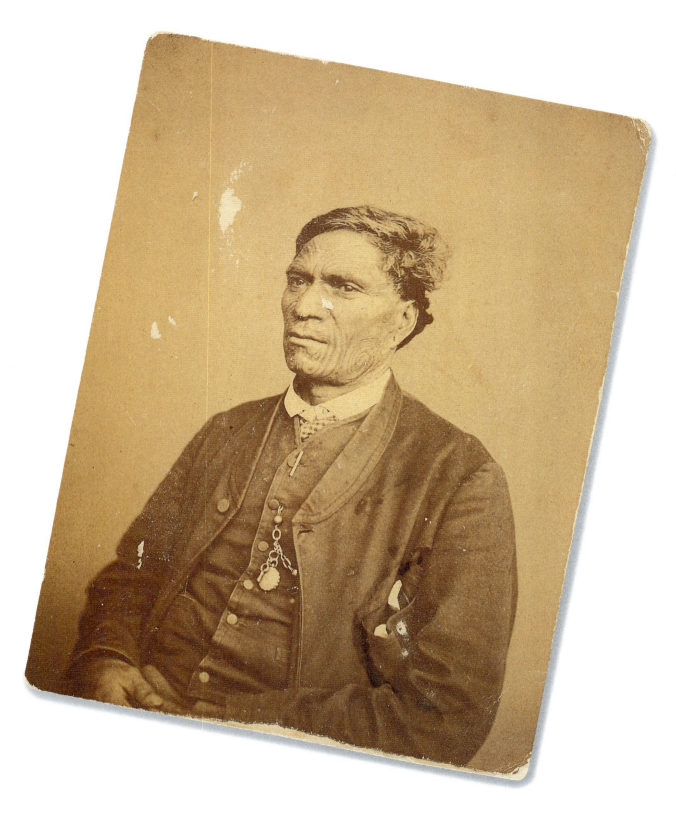

"Rawiri (David) Te Maire of Ngai Tahu and Ngati Kahungunu South Island." An important Maori of rank, he was an ordained Anglican minister and noted writer on Maori matters. He is also remembered for having political aspirations. In this photograph, he is seen dressed in fine European clothing of the period, complete with watch and fob dangling from his vest. A strange image showing a Maori living in both worlds – one European, the other Maori. Albumen photograph mounted on board circa 1860s.

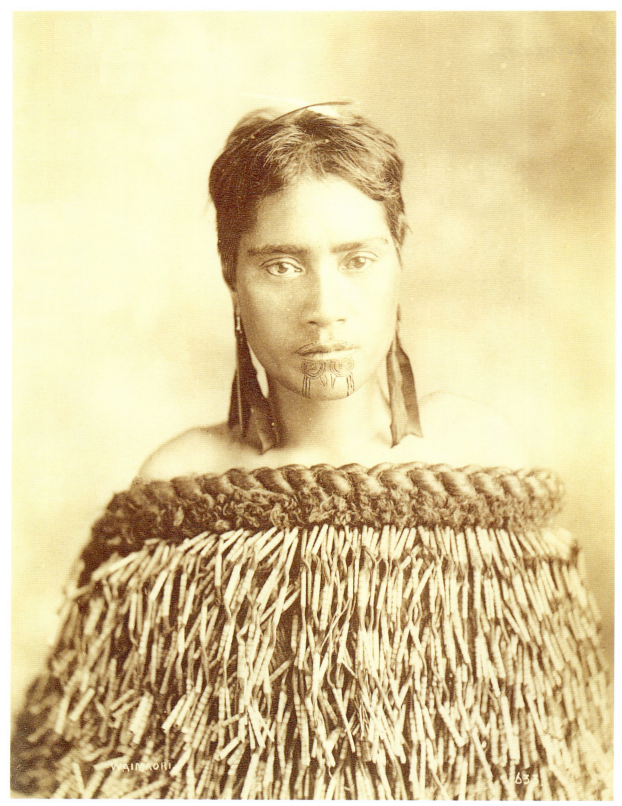

"Waimaori." A striking portrait of a woman of whose history we have no record. In this portrait, she appears to be in mourning with cropped hair and black ribbon earrings. Her chin and lip moko is a good example of the revival in women's tattoo that took place around 1875. Original albumen photograph mounted on board, photographer unknown. Circa 1870s.

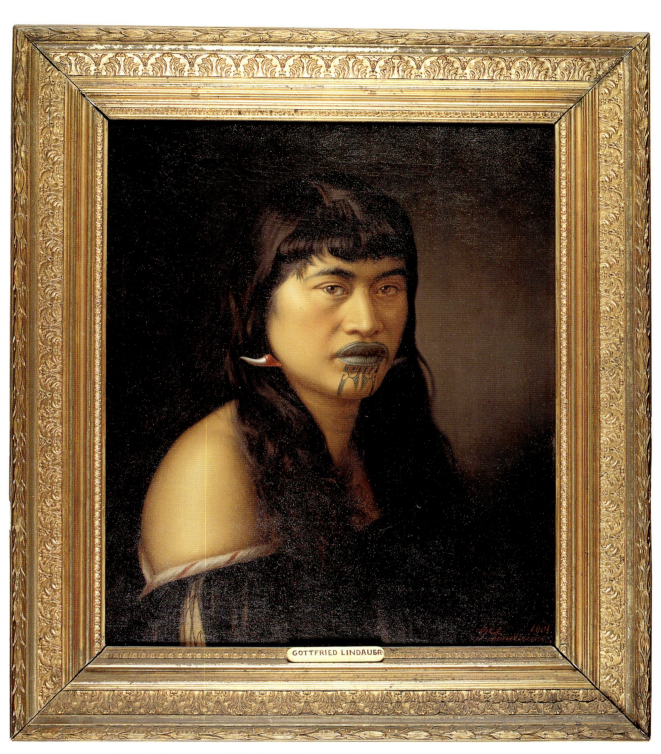

Original oil painting of "Hinekura of Te Reinga, Hawkes Bay, North Island" by Gottfried Lindauer.* According to Dr. D. R. Simmons in his book entitled *Maori Tattoo*,** he states, "she was a tapairu, a wahine ariki of the second line of Ngati Marumaru, Nga Herehere, Ngati Kahungunu and many other tribes. She came down by the male line on both her father's and her mother's sides shown by the "tongues" in the semi circles. The small spirals at the sides are the sign that she belongs to the second line." Signed and dated 1901.

*Gottfried Lindauer (1839-1926) a Bohemian by birth and one of New Zealand's greatest artists was best known for his Maori subject matter. For further information see the book entitled *Maori Paintings* by Gottfried Lindauer, edited by J.C. Graham, Auckland City Council Publishers, 1965.
**Published in 1989 by the Bush Press, Auckland, New Zealand.

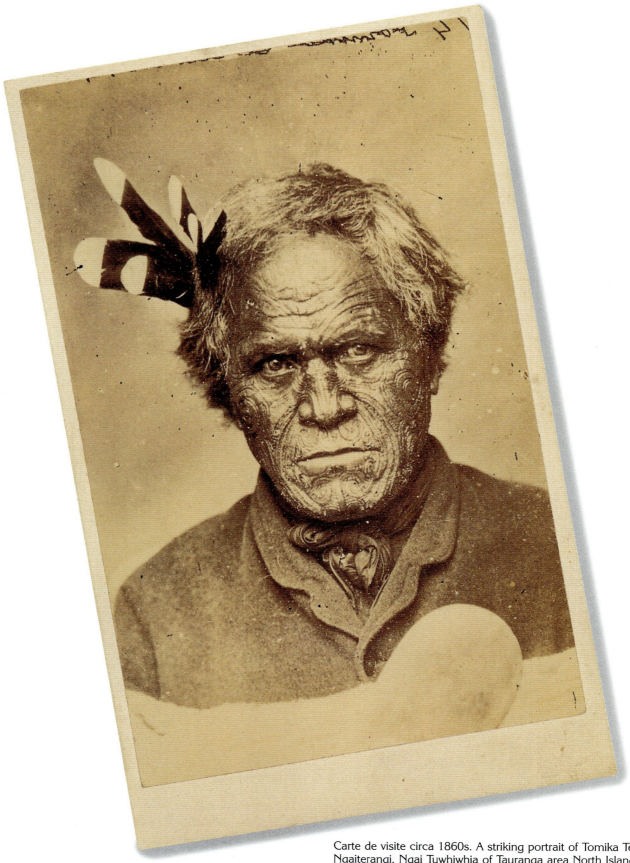

Carte de visite circa 1860s. A striking portrait of Tomika Te Mutu of Ngaiterangi, Ngai Tuwhiwhia of Tauranga area North Island. A chief primarily based in Motuhoa Island, he is shown here with a striking moko applied during the early part of the 19th century. Photographer unknown.

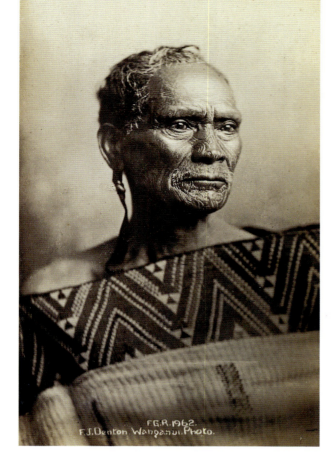

"Tangata, a chief of Te Atihau a Paparangi of Wanganui North Island." Very little if anything is known about this chief. A most imposing portrait, the chief is seen wearing a fine *kaitaka* flax cloak with a wide *taniko* border. From original postcard entitled "F.G.R. 1962, F.J. Denton, Wanganui Photo." Circa 1910.

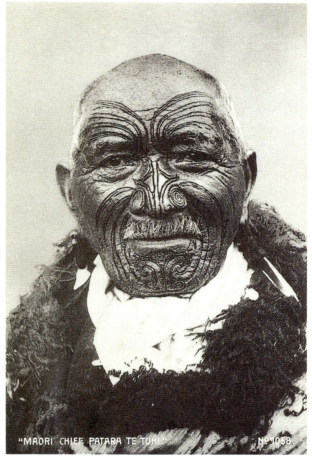

"Te Tuhi, Wiremu Patara chief of the Ngati Mahuta." Original postcard entitled "Maori Chief Patara Te Tuhi" published by W. Beattie and Co. Fine Art Publishers Auckland N.Z. circa 1910. A much more "Maori" portrait in style and dress. See page 85 for more information.

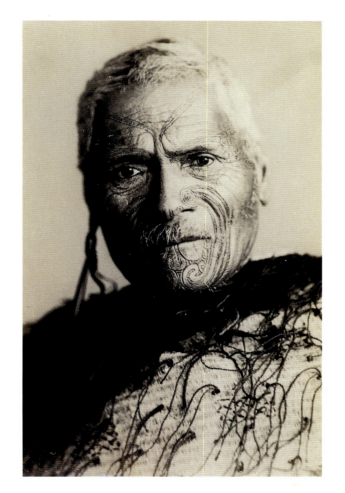

"Unidentified chief of the Te Ati Hau a Paparangi of the North Island." The chief depicted here is wearing a *korowai* class cloak. He appears to be from the Wanganui river area of the south west of the North Island. His forehead and nose moko is unusual. From original postcard hand-stamped on reverse "New Zealand Post Card" circa 1920.

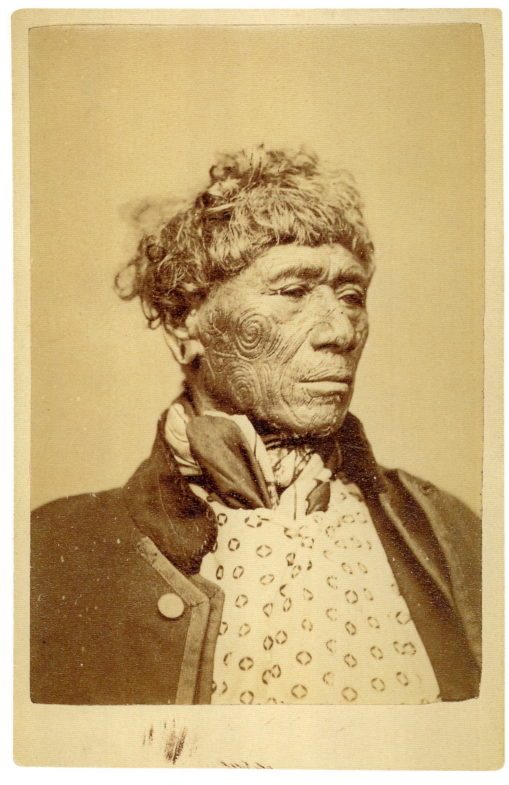

Carte de visite. This poignant image depicts an unidentified chief with full "chisel" moko. Photograph taken in 1860 by the American Photographic Company at the Kohimarama Conference.

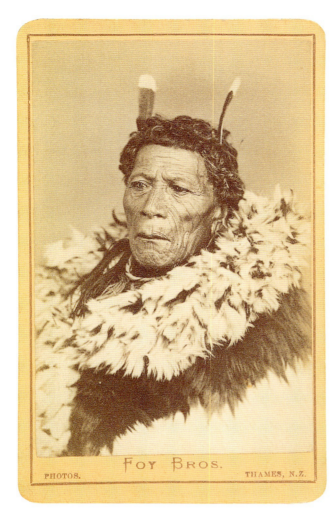

Carte de visite circa 1860's. This image depicts the high chief Ahirore of the Ngati Maru tribe in Hawkes Bay, North Island. Foy Brothers photographers, Thames.

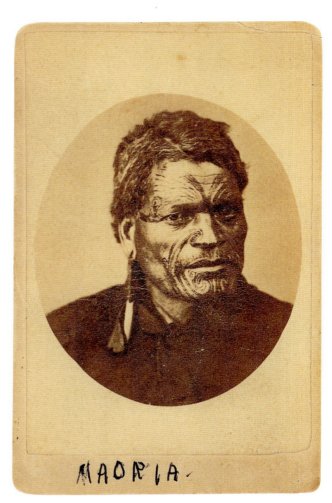

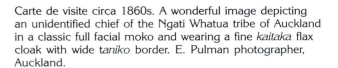

Carte de visite circa 1860s. A portrait of Maoria of Taranaki tribe and Te Atihau a Paparangi of the Wanganui River. He is best known for stopping the Maori rebels from attacking Wanganui township at Moutoa Island in the Maori Wars of 1863/1864. He fought with the British Forces and was considered a hero by the *pakeha*. Photographer unknown.

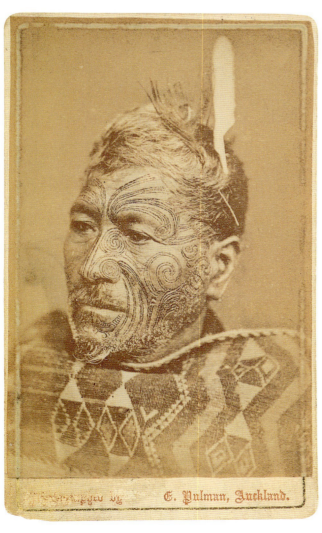

Carte de visite circa 1860s. A wonderful image depicting an unidentified chief of the Ngati Whatua tribe of Auckland in a classic full facial moko and wearing a fine *kaitaka* flax cloak with wide *taniko* border. E. Pulman photographer, Auckland.

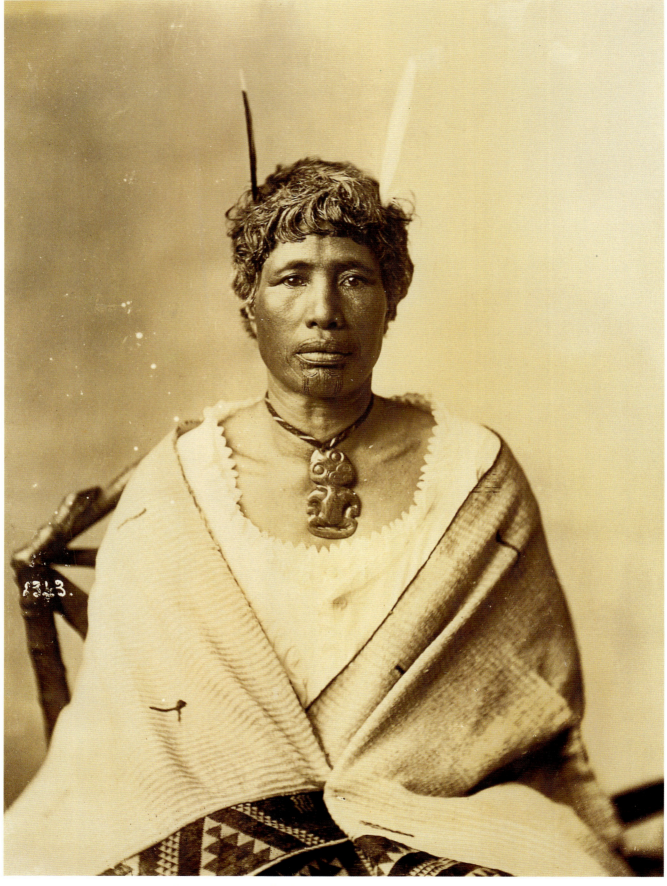

"Unknown Woman." This lady, possibly from the east coast of the North Island, is a good example of the revival in women's tattooing that took place around 1875. Here she is shown wearing her *hei tiki* and flax cloak posing for the photographer. Original albumen photograph, photographer unknown. Circa 1880s. Formerly in the collection of Elsdon Best and Dr. Terence Barrow.

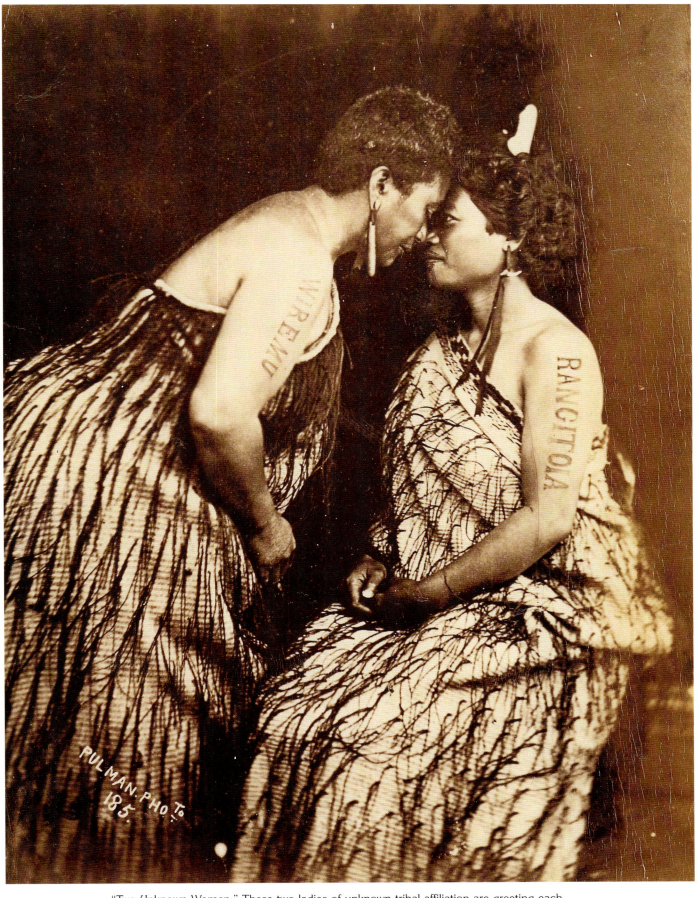

"Two Unknown Women." These two ladies of unknown tribal affiliation are greeting each other in the traditional *hongi* style. What makes this photo most interesting is that both women have tattoos on their arms (retouched by the photographer). The words are Wiremu and Rangitoia, presumably their baptismal names. This type of tattooing is thought to have originated with the missionaries – permanently marking their early converts. Original albumen photograph mounted on board, Pulman Photo #185. Circa 1880s.

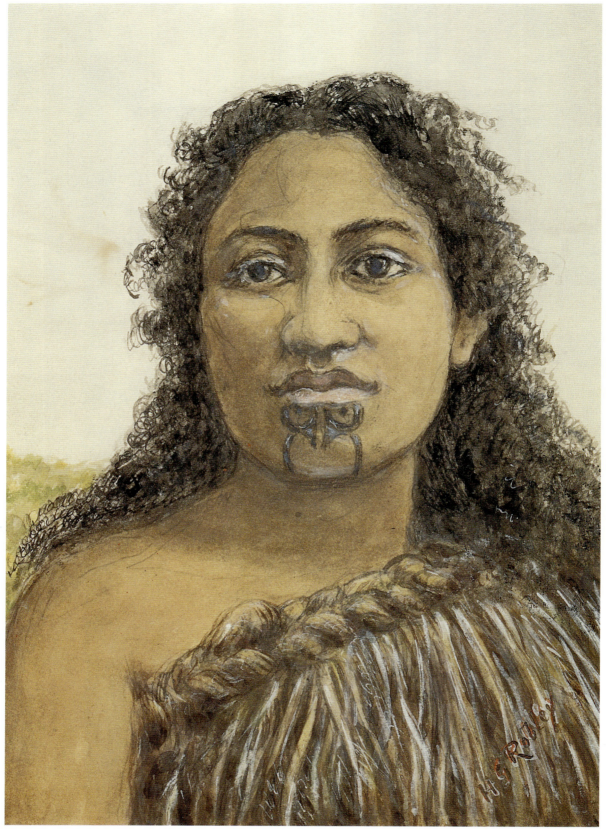

Original watercolor by General Horatio Gordon Robley. This picture depicting a woman of the Ngai Te Rangi tribe showing a classic chin tattoo was done during the Maori Wars in the 1860s. The design of the two incurving spirals suggests to some that she may have been the first born of her family.

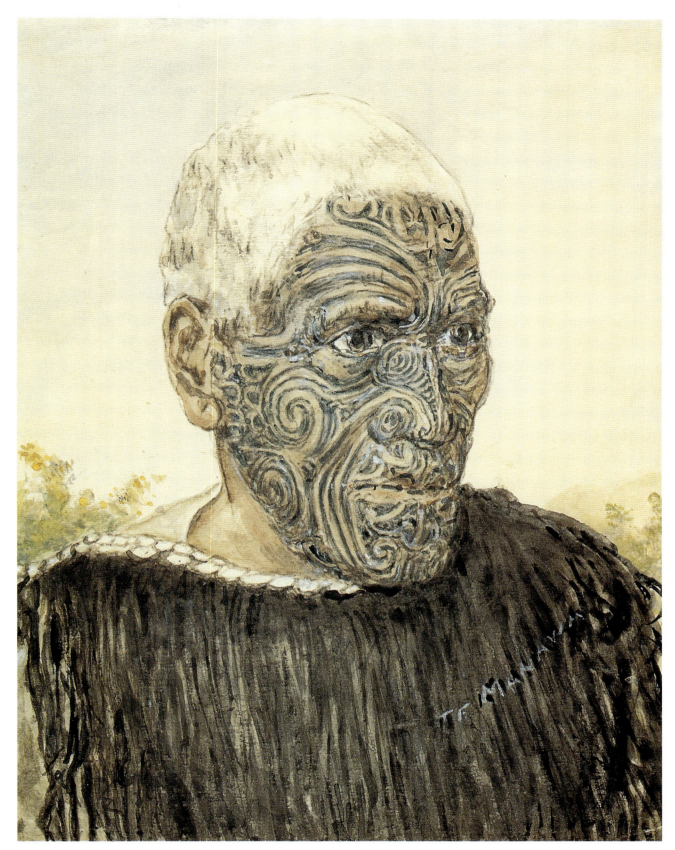

Original watercolor by Major General Horatio Gordon Robley. In this portrait, Wi Te Manewha of Ngati Raukawa is shown with tight spirals on his nose, possibly indicating that he was a *pukorero*, an orator, while the design beside his ear identifies him as a carver for the *taiopuru* (paramount chief). He fought in the battle of the Kuititanga between the Ngati Ruakawa and the Ngati Awa on the beach in Waikanae and is remembered as a great warrior. Both sides suffered terribly in this battle and the Maori on both sides agreed to have the surgeon from the British ship *Tory* land to attend the wounded.

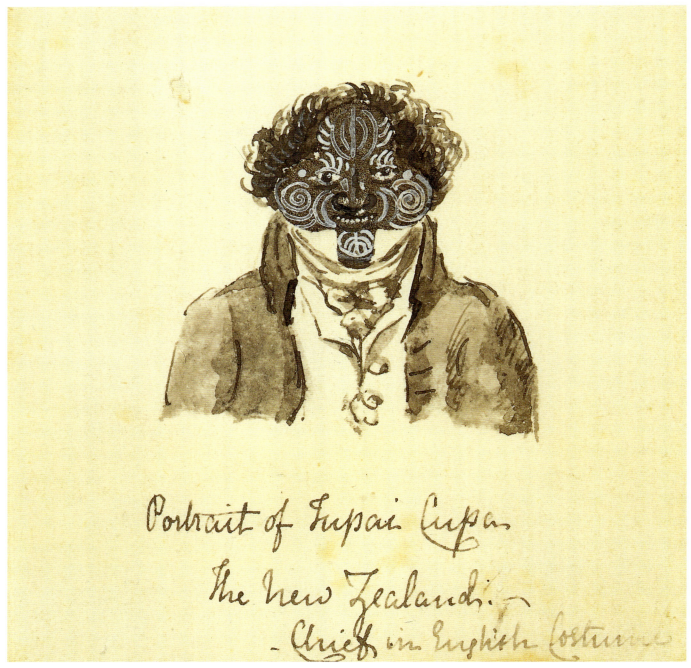

"Te Pehi Kupe paramount chief of the Ngati Toa at Porirua North Island." A very powerful chief during the "musket wars." In 1816 he went to England to buy muskets for his war chief Te Rauparaha. In 1828 he was killed at Onawe *pa* on the Bank's Peninsula. In 1830 Te Rauparaha took terrible revenge on the *pa* and gave the chief of the *pa* to Te Pehi Kupe's widows. The chief died three days later. The revenge party traveled on a European ship whose captain was later arrested and his ship confiscated when he reached Sydney, Australia. From original drawing done in London, presumably in 1816 by an anonymous artist. This rare portrait was found in an early album of calling cards from the late 18th and early 19th centuries - among the other notable items was the calling card of the Tahitian Omai of Captain Cook's Voyages fame.

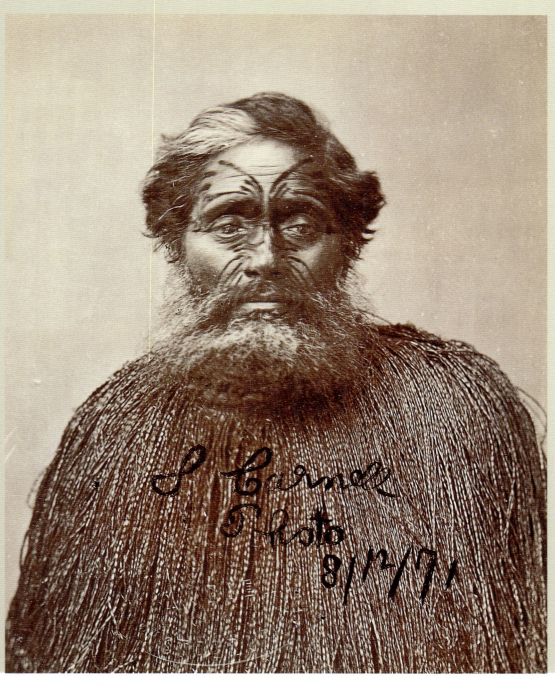

"Te Rau, Kereopa (Cleophas) of the Ngati Rangiwewehi of the Te Arawa, North Island." A noted warrior and Pai Marire leader, he represents a tragic figure in the New Zealand wars and insurgencies of the period. Baptized in the 1840s by the Catholic Church, he is believed to have served as a policeman in Auckland in the 1850s. In the early 1860s, he fought in the King's forces in Waikato. Government forces at Rangiaowhia killed his wife and children on February 21, 1864, and the following day he saw his sister killed at Hairini, a defensive position just west of Rangiaowhia. After the defeat of the King movement forces, he joined the new religion of Te Ua Haumene. Shortly after this he was instructed by Te Ua to go as an emissary to the tribes on the east coast. He was told along with Patara to preach the Pai Marire faith in the districts they passed through and to go in peace. Ignoring this, Kereopa demanded that a European be given up to him at Otipa, a settlement on the lower Rangitaiki River, and that a Catholic priest be given up to him at Whakatane. Infuriated, he seized the missionary C. S. Volkner at Opotiki, Gisborne District, and ritually killed him on March 2, 1865. Upon this act, Kereopa swallowed his eyes and drank his blood from the church chalice. One eye he called the parliament the other the Queen and the British law. Although this act outraged Europeans, in Maori culture to perform such an indignity to the head of an enemy conferred additional *mana*. He had further skirmishes with the Ngati Manaw, Ngati Rangitihi, and the Government troops throughout the next several years and earned the name Kaiwhatu, eye eater, after swallowing three additional Ngati Manawa warriors' eyes, again in a ritualistic form. On December 21, 1871, Kereopa finally stood trial after he was captured after several unfortunate turns of events. Kereopa was convicted of the murder by an eyewitness who testified that he saw him among the congregation members who escorted Volkner to the tree for hanging. Mother Mary Aubert, of Father Reigners' mission at Napier, stayed with Kereopa his last night. He was hanged on January 5, 1872. This disturbing photograph, taken shortly before being captured, gives the feeling of a "caged animal." Original photograph with retouched moko by S. Carnell, Napier. Photographer's name in blind-stamp seal along with inscription on front reading "S. Carnell Photo 8/12/74." Formerly in the collection of Elsdon Best and Dr. Terence Barrow.

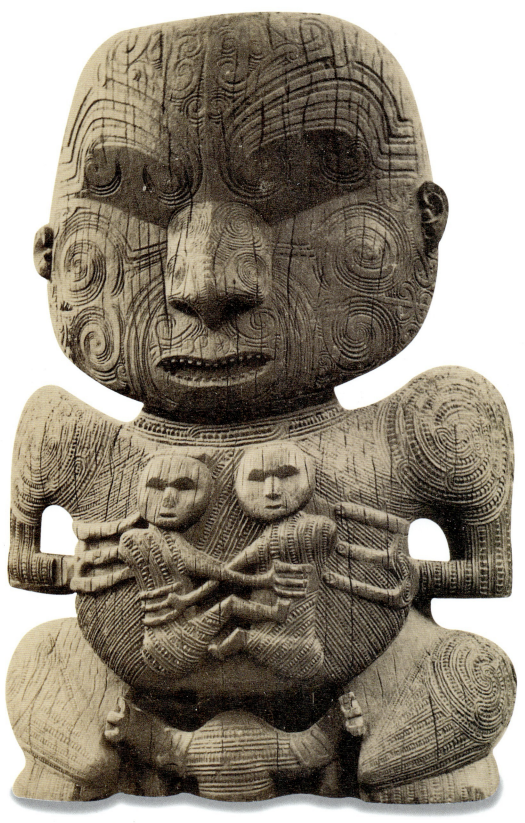

Large figure from the gateway of a *pa* (village) that stood at Te Ngae on Lake Rotorua in the early part of the 19th century. The figure topped a gateway that was over 15 feet high, the lower part being broken off and lost. The main figure, which is heavily tattooed, represents a chief of the Ngati Whakaue tribe named Pukaki with his wife and two children. The main chiefly figure shows a classic moko tattoo of the Arawa people. The arms and legs are likewise decorated in classic Arawa spirals. Actual size of fragment depicted is 6 feet 5-1/8 inches in height. From original postcard printed in Edinburgh, Scotland circa 1910. Piece is now housed in Auckland Institute and Museum, Auckland, New Zealand.

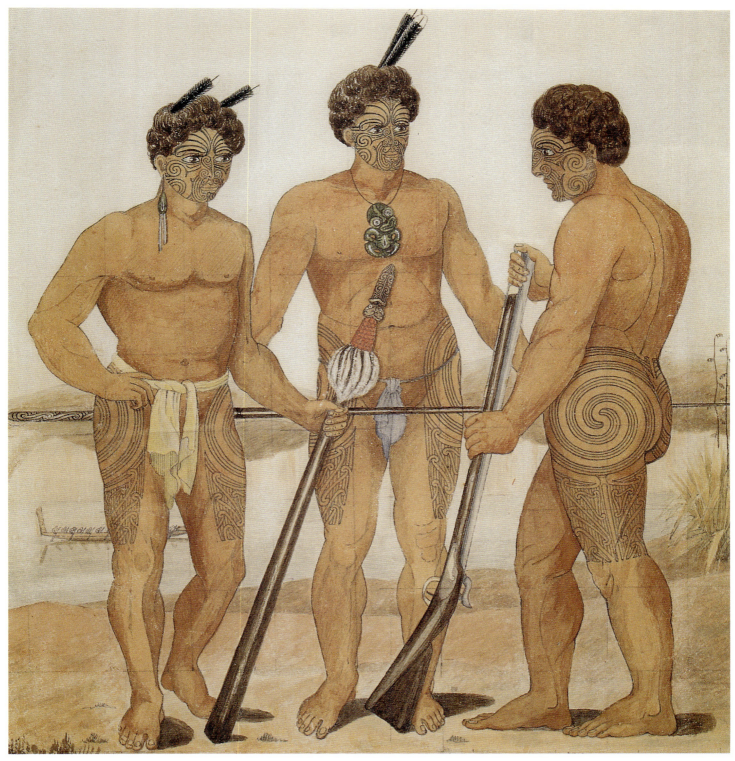

Original watercolor by Joseph Jenner Merrett.* The hunchbacked person to the right in this powerful picture has a *koru* loop going up and down by his ear. He is a *tohunga* of the upper and lower way with his moko identifying him as Te Wairoa, a paramount chief of the Tuhoe and Taranaki tribes. This portrait also shows a good example of buttock tattoo prevalent in some areas at this time. The center man is of a higher rank with a forehead design and can be identified as Waaka Putere of Ngat Kahungunu and Tuwharetoa. Here he is depicted with a jade *hei tiki* around his neck. The man holding the *taiaha* is Tainui Hawea of Taranaki and Tuhoe; he has five forehead rays on one side, six on the other.

*J.J. Merrett (1816-1854) was a surveyor who contributed enormously to the record of New Zealand around the mid-19th century. He was well known for recording the Maori people and culture. His Maori paintings illustrate, among others, A.S. Thomson's *The Story of New Zealand*, 1859. He was an eyewitness to numerous important historical events including the famous Maori feast held near Auckland in 1844 that lasted over a week, with over 4,000 native people in attendance.

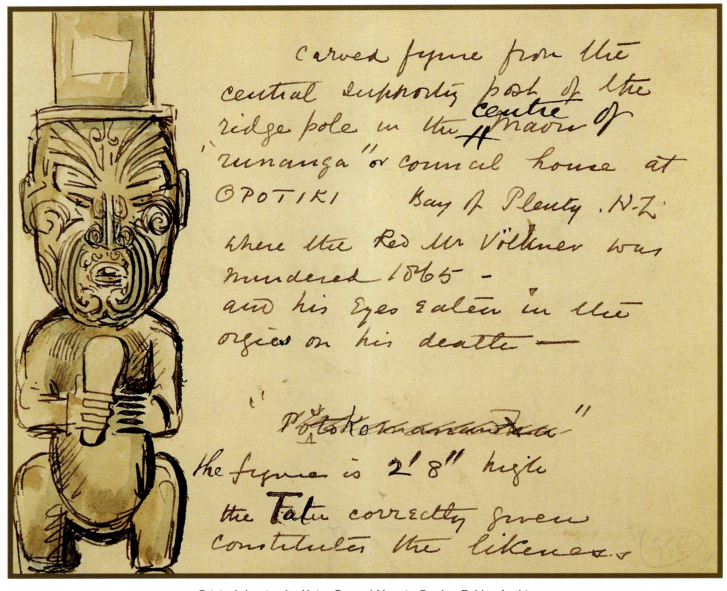

Original drawing by Major General Horatio Gordon Robley. In this picture, a *pou tokomanawa* is depicted with full moko. Inscribed as follows: "carved from the central supporting post of the ridge pole in the council house at Opotiki Bay of Plenty, N.Z. where the Rev. Mr Volkner was murdered in 1865 and his eyes eaten in the orgies on his death – the figure is 2'8" high the TATU correctly given contributes the likeness." Circa late 1860s.

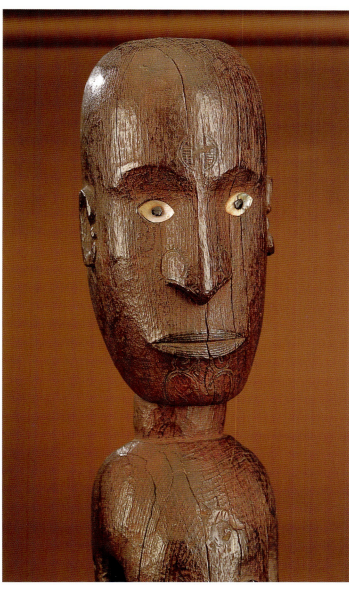
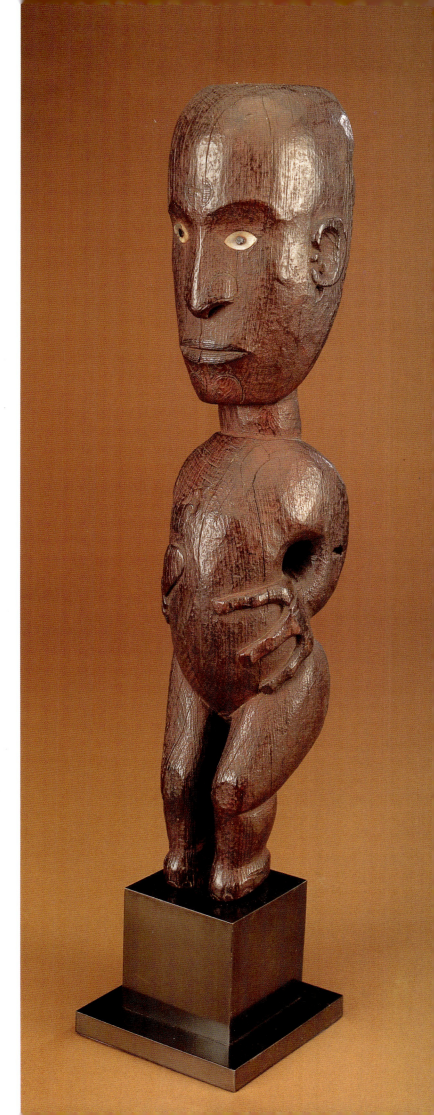

"*Pou tokomanawa*" or house post sculpture. This rare figure has been cut away from a post that supported the middle portion of a house ridge-beam. According to Dr. D. R. Simmons,* "the female figure holds a jade club in her left hand indicating a female chief."** He further states: "that the moko, which is very unusual, suggests by the forehead design that she belonged to the third line and was of Ngati descent. The lines on her lips also confirm this. The spiral on the nose is that of a *tapu* or sacred person who also trained as a warrior and perhaps a servitor to a person of a very high rank. The chin tattoo is that of a lady who is the eldest daughter on both mother's and father's sides, with pendants in circles. The lowest lines curve, then go down to under the chin line; this is a sign, again, that she was the servitor of a high female chief, a bit like a lady in waiting or bodyguard to the Queen. Stylistically this could fit quite nicely into the Ngati Tuwharetoa corpus for a house that was built for a chief in the Taupo area of the central North Island. Being a person of high rank in her own right, it is possible that this figure could represent Hinemoa, a chieftaness named after her famous ancestor Hinemoa who featured in the Rotorua love story of Hinemoa and Tutanekai. This later Hinemoa of Ngati Puhara sub-tribe of Tuwharetoa lived some eight generations ago. Wood and paua shell with traces of red "barn" paint." Height: 17-3/4 inches. Circa 1830/1850.
*Personal communication, 1993
**These small jade clubs "*mere pounamu*" are much rarer than the usual jade clubs encountered and were specially balanced for left-hand use only.

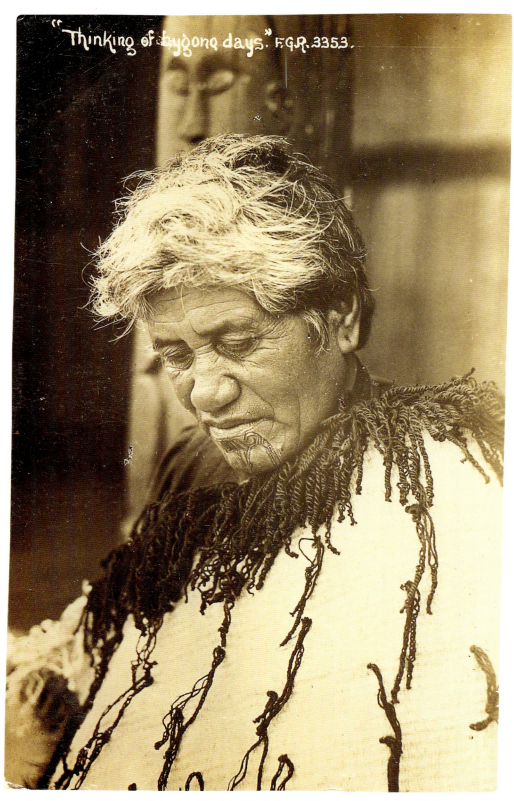

"Te Ahinata Te Rangi Tautini, a chieftaness of the Tuhourangi tribe of Te Arawa, North Island." Also known as "Kapikapi." This photo was originally taken by John Pringle in the early part of the 20th century. She died about 1920 and was reputed to be 136 years old at the time of her death. She was a favorite of artist Charles F. Goldie and was the subject matter of many of his paintings. According to some, her chin tattoo and spirals on her nose indicated she was a lady in waiting to a chief of high rank, her own rank being notable as well. In this photograph, the photographer has retouched the chin tattoo. From original photo postcard entitled "Thinking of Bygone Days" F.G.R. #3353. Circa 1915.

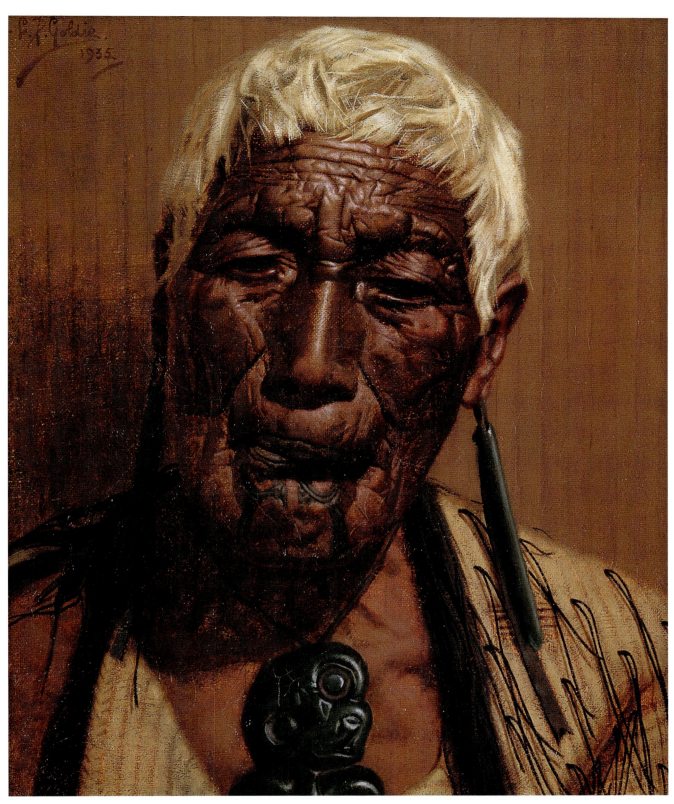

Original oil painting of "Mere Werohia" by Charles F. Goldie.* A noted chieftaness of the Rotorua District, she was a favorite subject of the artist and he painted her numerous times. In this remarkable portrait a great sadness comes forth. An important picture for the student of tattoo as it shows - with "photo-like" accuracy - a good example of mid-19th century grooved chisel tattoo work. Signed and dated 1935 with inscription on reverse: "A chieftaness of the Ngati te Roro te Rangi Hapu of the Ngatiwhakane Tribe, Rotorua."

*Charles F. Goldie (1870-1947) is considered - along with Lindauer - one of two of the greatest artists ever to paint the Maori people. For more information on Maori portraits done by this artist see the book entitled *Goldie* by Roger Blackley, Auckland Art Gallery, 1997.

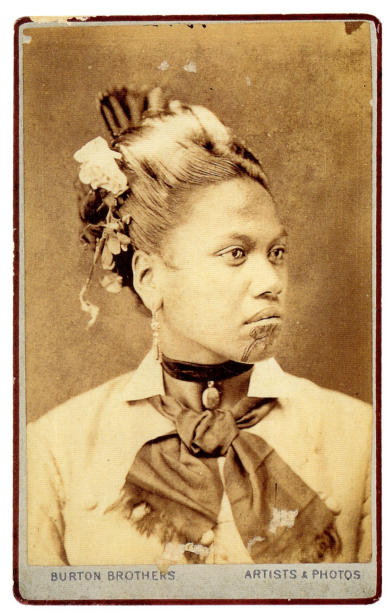

Carte de visite. An unknown woman who by her moko appears to be the eldest child of a chief who was closely related to a paramount line, if the reading of here tattoo is correct. She appears also to be from the Te Atiawa of Taranaki area of the North Island. Image marked on mount "Burton Brothers Artists and Photos." Circa 1870s.

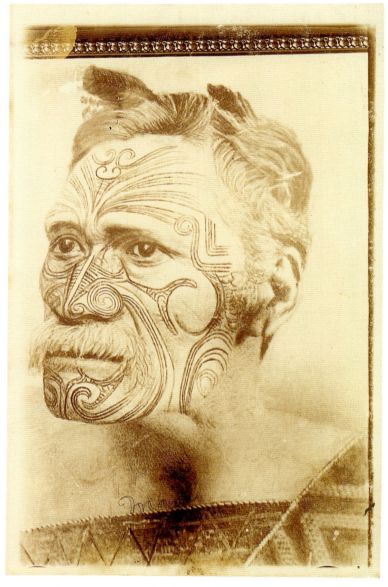

"Kewene Te Haho of Ngati Naho, Ngati Whawhakia of Waikato, North Island." A paramount chief, according to Dr. D. R. Simmons,* who "belonged to a line that had died out and was started again from the collateral line, hence the curious moko designs on his cheek." His tribe is well known as being neutral in the fight between the Europeans and Waikato Maori; hence, even to this day, his people are sometimes called traitors by other Waikato tribes. In this curious photo, the photographer has retouched the moko, inking over the original photograph. From original real postcard, unmarked, circa 1905.
*Personal communication, 1998.

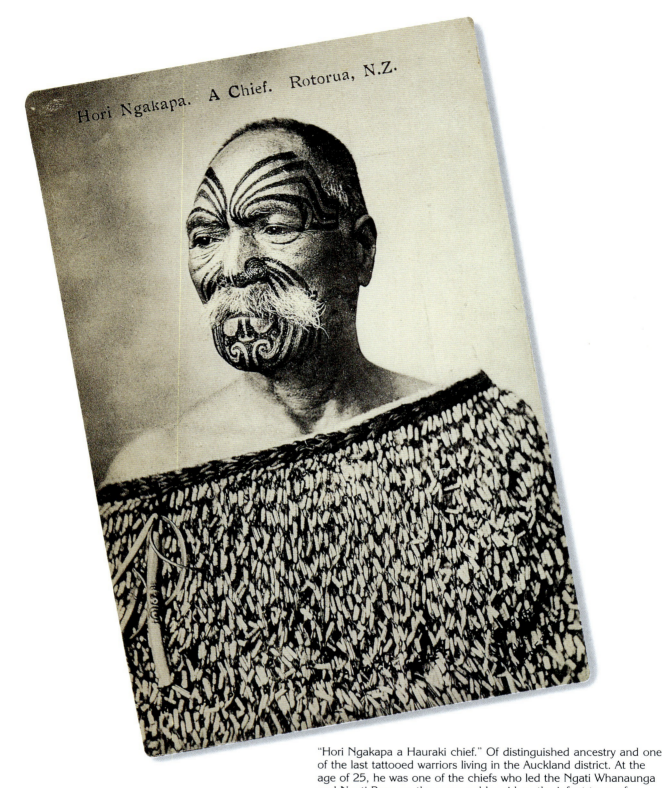

"Hori Ngakapa a Hauraki chief." Of distinguished ancestry and one of the last tattooed warriors living in the Auckland district. At the age of 25, he was one of the chiefs who led the Ngati Whanaunga and Ngati Paoa on the memorable raid on the infant town of Auckland in 1851. Then in 1863, he led a large party of Ngati Whanaunga to the defense of Rangiriri *pa*. The British did not capture him during the fall of Rangiriri as he escaped with some of his followers by swimming across the lake to safety. He then went on to Ngaruawahia the Maori capital, and then to Paterangi, where he was one of those who garrisoned the strongly fortified Kingitie *pa*. At the end of the war in 1864 he returned home to the shores of Hauraki Gulf where he cooperated fully with the government, helping open the lands of the area for gold mining. In this striking photographic portrait, his moko has been retouched and differs widely from the painting commissioned in 1874 by the artist Gottfried Lindauer. In this photo, far fewer forehead lines are noticeable. From original postcard entitled "Hori Ngakapa – A Chief, Rotorua, N.Z." Published by Isles, Rotorua.

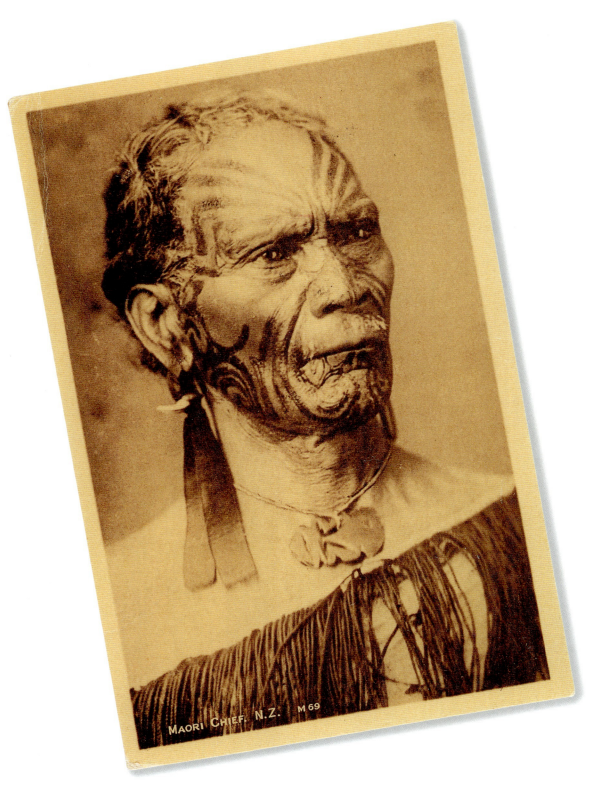

"Kamareira Te Hau Takiri Wharepapa of Ngati Horahia, Nga Titoki, Ngapuhi of Northland, North Island." A Maori chief of note, having traveled to England in 1863, he had a royal audience with Queen Victoria. While in England with other notable chiefs, he married an English woman, which caused quite a stir in prudish Victorian society. Today, he has many descendants living in New Zealand, some having married into Maori families, others into prominent *pakeha* families. In this striking portrait he is shown in a defiant pose with a moko that has been prominently exaggerated, the photographer using black paint or some other form of enhancement. This is an interesting image, which, when examined closely, appears quite unsettling with the *hei tiki* pendant deliberately turned away from the viewer, very possibly so the *mana* of the piece would not be affected by the photograph. From original postcard entitled "Maori Chief N.Z.," J.D. Kemp Quality Photographers. Circa 1920/1930.

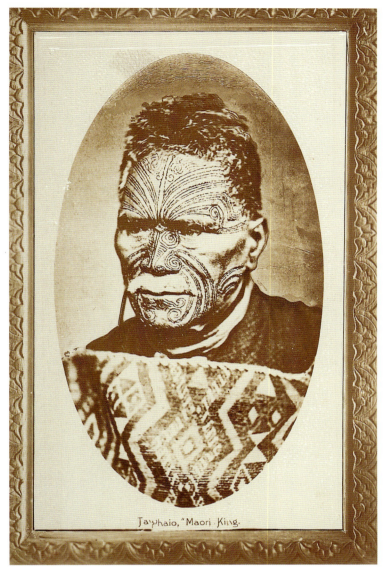

"Tawhaio, Maori King." Embossed border postcard printed in Britain and numbered 315 circa 1910. Photo with moko retouched showing Tawahaio in a rather defiant pose near the end of his illustrious life.

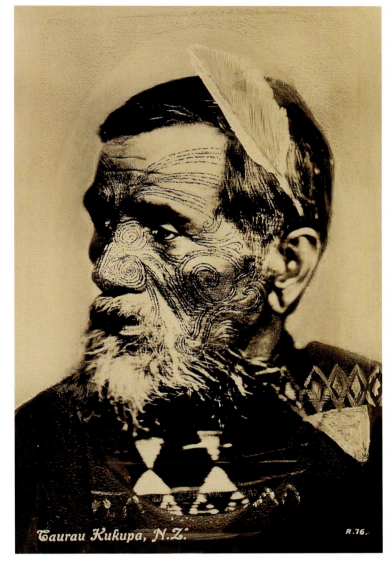

"Taurau Kukupa chief of the Te Parawhau, of Whangarei North Island." A notable Maori leader, he was described as "tall and commanding" by an early missionary. He succeeded his famous brother Te Tirarau Kukupa upon his death in 1882. He is most noted as an advocate of his people. Although this photograph appears to have been retouched to enhance the moko, it shows a classic series of spiral designs done in the early part of the 19th century. From original postcard entitled "Taurau Kukupa, N.Z." Tanner Bros. Ltd. Maoriland Photographic series – Wellington N.Z. circa 1910.

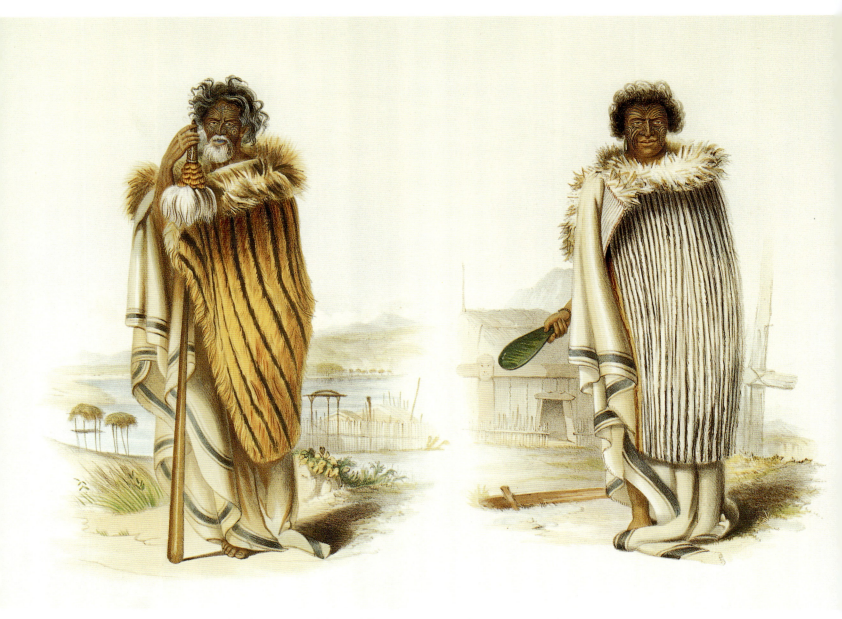

"Muriwenua and Kahawai." Drawn from life by George Angas, 1844. At the time of this drawing, Muriwhenua was the oldest living chief from Aotea, a harbor on the West Coast of the North Island. He belonged to the Nga Te Pare or Ngati Pari tribe of Waingaroa. In this drawing, he has seven forehead rays on one side and six on the other. The forehead decoration suggests a *kohere* or paramount chief. According to Angas, he was a celebrated warrior who "had unusual powers of sorcery" and Kahawai "was a chief of the Nga ti hinetu tribe residing among his people at Ngahuruhuru in the Waipa district." Original lithograph from two-volume set published in 1846 entitled *The New Zealanders Illustrated* by George French Angas.

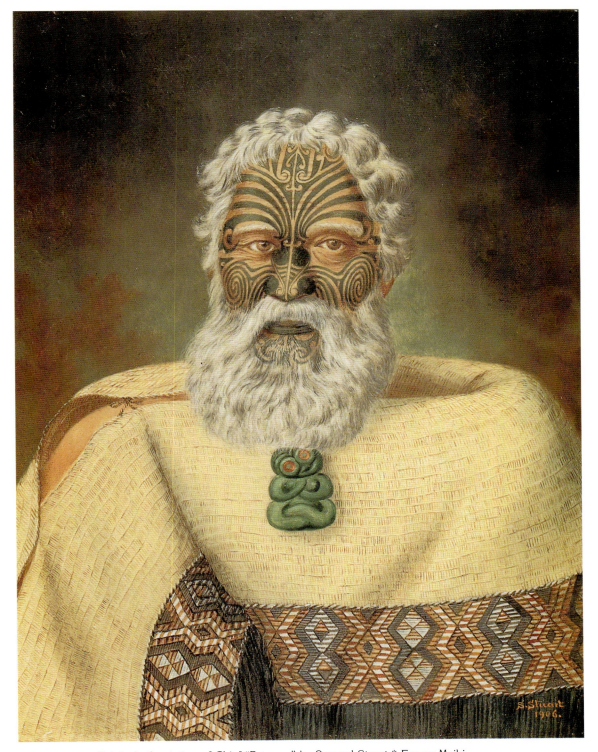

Original oil painting of Chief "Patuone" by Samuel Stuart.* Eruera Maihi Patuone was a famous and benevolent chief of the Ngapuhi tribe and elder brother of the celebrated Tamati Waka Nene. Patuone came from a long line of noble ancestors and was one of the last living Maori to recall seeing Captain Cook's ship *Endeavour* at Cape Brett, Bay of Islands. He was a noted warrior and comrade-in-arms of Hongi Hika even though he never lifted a hand against the newly arrived Europeans. He often served as a mediator between various hostile parties and early missionaries who would often ask for his assistance. He was well over 100 years old when he died in 1872. A monument was erected over his grave: "To the memory of Patuone the Peacemaker." Looking at his moko, some people have speculated that it shows his mother was on the second line of the Ngapuhi and has pledged protection to the *taiopuru*. Signed and dated 1906.

*Samuel Stuart (1855-1920), little is known about this New Zealand artist, being most active in the years 1877-1906. For further information see the book entitled *Two Hundred Years of New Zealand Painting by Gil Docking*, David Bateman Publishers, Auckland, 1990.

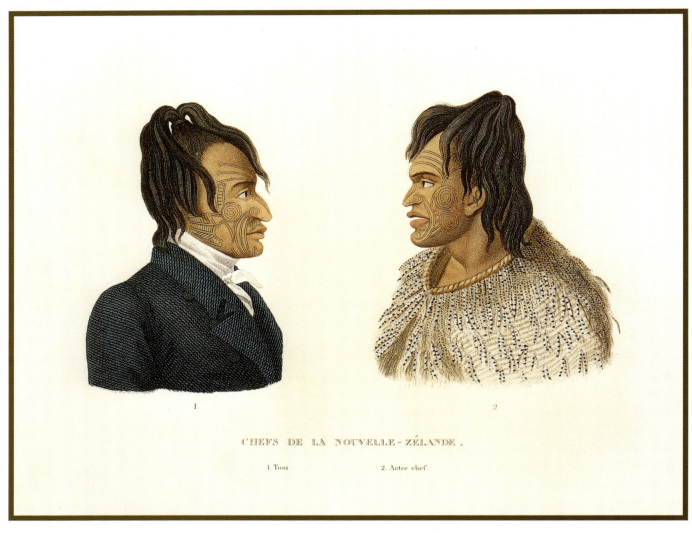

"Chefs De La Nouvelle – Zelande." Original lithograph by French artist Jules Le Jeune, who drew this portrait in 1824.*
In this print, Toui of Kahouwera *pa* in the Bay of Islands is depicted dressed in European finery. An important paramount chief, his lineage is confirmed in his striking moko. Based upon some interpretations in "reading" moko, the other chief, depicted in more traditional garb, has design elements showing his *mana* as a warrior. In a sad note, Toui was killed shortly after his portrait was drawn and Kahouwera sacked.
*Jules Le Jeune was the official artist of Captain Louis Isidore Duperrey's ship the *Coquille,* which circumnavigated the world in 1822-1825 on behalf of France.

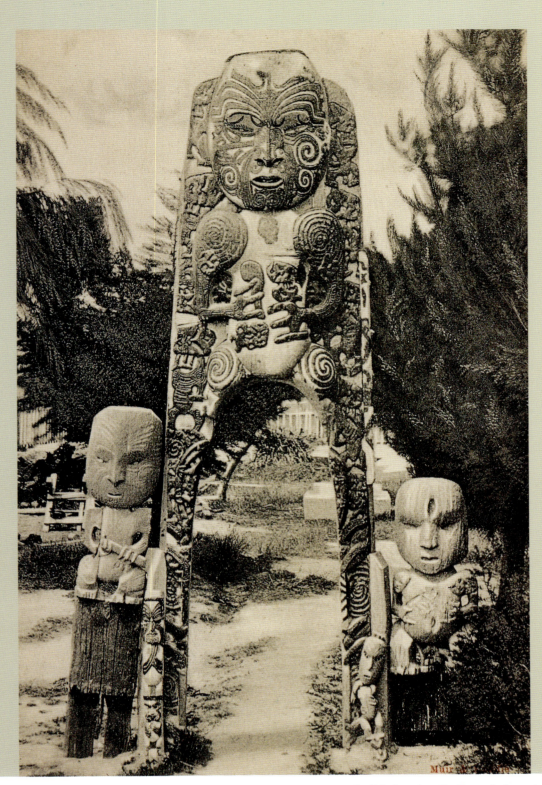

Famous gateway of Pukeroa *pa* (village). This *waharoa* (gateway) was located on the foreshore of Lake Rotorua and was the main entrance to this very impressive palisaded village and was standing until 1845. Possibly carved in the early 19th century, Pukeroa was one of the principal villages of the Ngati Whakaue tribe. The male figure depicted in this carving is shown with a classic Arawa moko. In Arawa moko, the father's side is the right-hand side of the face and the mother's the left. This according to Dr. D. R. Simmons who further states "that instead of a tribal spiral for his father, Tutanekai (depicted on this carving) has the symbol of an arikinui as his father, his forehead design is that of Kaitahutahu arikinui - the rank given him by Whakaue. Tutanekai was the son of Tuwharetoa by Whakaue's wife; Tutanekai's moko indicates that he was a person of ability, but the mere fact of him having it was due to the greatness of mind of Whakaue himself."* The original face of this carving was painted white with black tattoo. The body was also white except for the shoulders and arms, which were painted red. A large and impressive masterwork of Maori sculpture measuring over 16 feet high. From original postcard issued by Muir and Moodie, Dunedin circa 1910. Sculpture is now housed in Auckland Institute and Museum, Auckland, New Zealand.

The Art of Maori Tattoo by Dr. D. R. Simmons, published in 1986 by Reed Methuen publishers of Auckland, New Zealand.

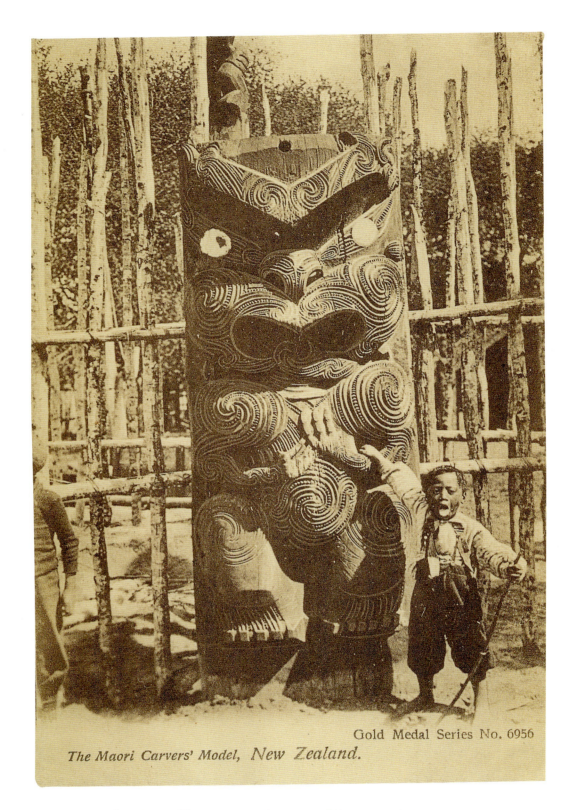

Gold Medal Series No. 6956
The Maori Carvers' Model, New Zealand.

46

Interior panel from tribal meeting house. This *poupou* depicts a male ancestral figure and is done in the classic steel tool era of the Gisborne carving tradition. Moko covers virtually the entire figure. The sculpture depicted would have measured approximately four feet high. Location of figure is presently unknown to author. An interesting and rather tragic item to be noted in this view is the Maori child doing the so-called "penny-*haka*" (a *haka* performed for money to amuse the European tourists). Views like this contributed to the image of the Maori people as simpletons. From original postcard published as Gold Medal Series #6956 Christchurch, New Zealand circa 1910.

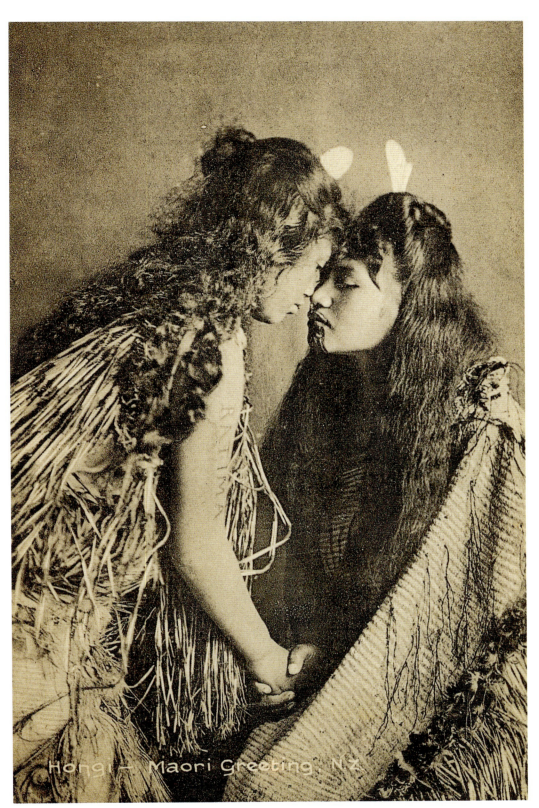

"Two Unknown Arawa Ladies." What makes this highly charged image most unusual is the word "Ratima" tattooed on the arm of one lady. This custom of tattooing a word or phrase on the body probably originated with the missionaries who devised a way of marking every convert they baptized. The word depicted here originated with the Church Missionary Society. In this image, the two ladies are greeting each other in typical fashion, but in reality this image portrayed a much more "erotic exotic" feeling. Photographers of this time period knew this type of image would sell, as the South Seas were viewed as an erotic haven and images like this perpetuated the "Myth of the South Seas." From original postcard entitled "Hongi – Maori Greeting, N.Z." published by Iles Rotorua. Circa 1910.

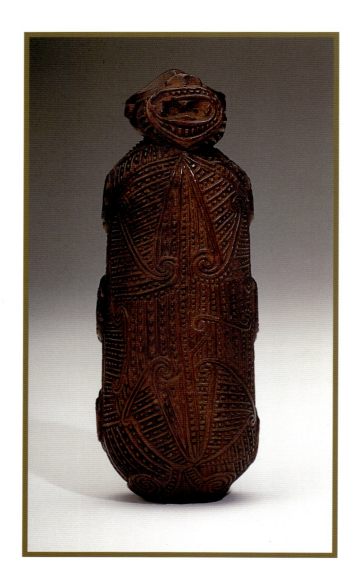

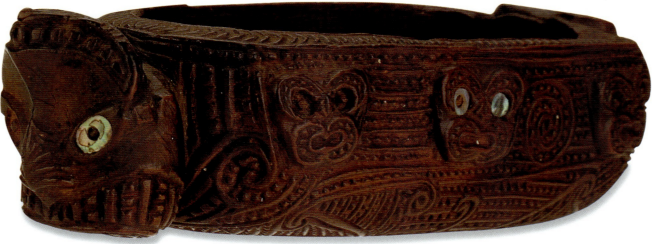

Pigment dish? A rare and unique item possibly used either for the red ocherous cosmetic powder known as *kokowai* or the black pigment of tattoo artistry. Stone carved of dense *kauri* wood in the East Coast-style of the North Island. The shape of this unusual item relates closely to the bone chests of the Maori. The underside is carved in an abstract human form motif. Traces of *Paua* shell inlay. 18th century. Length: 6-5/8 inches. Formerly in the Konietzko Collection, Hamburg, Germany.

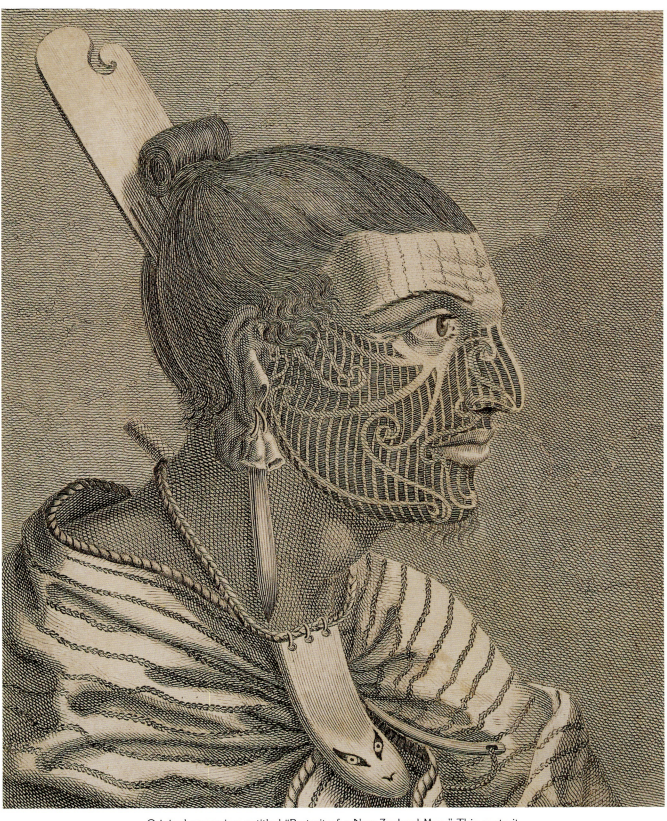

Original engraving entitled "Portrait of a New Zealand Man." This portrait is without a doubt the most famous depiction of a Maori person ever done. Drawn by Sydney Parkinson, artist with Captain Cook on his first voyage in 1769-1770, this picture represents a portrait of one of the chiefs of the southern side of the Turanganui inlet at Gisborne. The forehead rays are in groups of three as are the mouth rays. Also on the cheek there are large spirals with minor secondary spirals on the jaw lines. The hair is tied up in the fashion of the day, a *tikitiki* topknot. The tattoo suggests that he is from the Ngati Porou. Circa 1784.

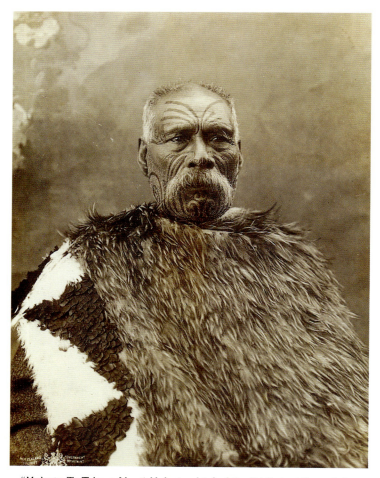

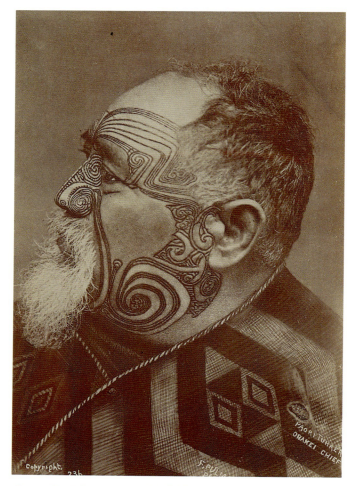

"Mahuta Te Teko a Ngati Mahuta chief of the Waikato tribes of the North Island." A cousin of King Tawahaio, he was one of the last tattooed men surviving in New Zealand at the time artist Charles F. Goldie painted him. At that time, many older important Maori men refused to be photographed or painted, being afraid their sacred *mana* would somehow be harmed. Goldie painted Mahuta Te Toko and described the event as follows: "I conveyed a studio for the purpose of the portrait; we very carefully heightened his handsome moko with black paint; with the result that when he looked in the mirror he was so delighted that he declared he would not wash his face for a month; his youth had been reknewed; he looked as if he had just been tattooed (without pain this time) and colored with the black Ngarehu pigment from the soot of burning kauri gum."*
From original postcard entitled "Mahuta Te Teko Maori Chief, N.Z. – Tourist Series #1." Published by Frank Duncan and Co. Ltd, Auckland, N.Z. Circa 1910.
Goldie by Roger Blackley, Auckland Art Gallery, 1997.

"Paora (Paul) Tuhaere chief of Te Taou section of Ngati Whatua ki Orakei Auckland, North Island." One of the most prominent chiefs of Auckland District, he was a favorite with photographers and artists. His tribe sold the land on which the town of Auckland was established. In this photograph, the photographer retouched the moko to overemphasize it, making it much more saleable in the tourist market. Original albumen photograph by F. Pulman copyright #236 circa 1890s.

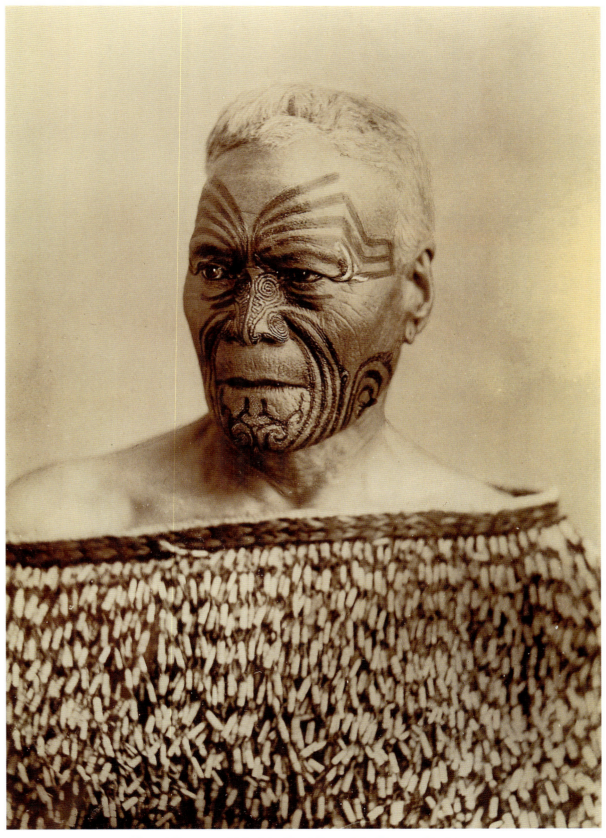

"Tuterei Karewa a chief of the Ngati Maru of the Thames District, North Island." A superb portrait depicting a stronger-than-usual moko highlighted by the photographer with the use of black paint or some other substance. Here he is dressed in a fine *pihepihe* shoulder cape with cylindrical tags of flax. Original albumen photograph by Isles #108 circa 1890s.

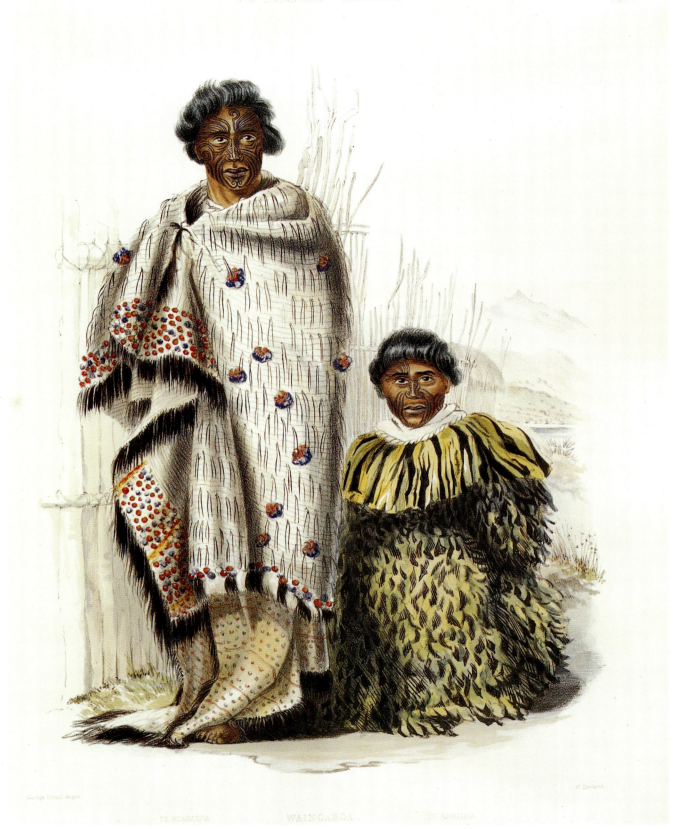

"Te Awaitaia and Te Moanaroa Waingaroa." Drawn from life by George Angas, 1844. Te Awaitaia was the chief of Ngati Mahanga. He is most noted for leading a raiding party into Taranaki in 1822 and for later important battles waged against the Ngapuhi. His most important line of descent came through his father, Te Kata, which is shown on the left forehead by the sign of a paramount chief, while his mother was of lesser rank. This suggests that his father was of *taiopuru* lineage. The rest of the moko suggests a chief of a sub-tribe derived from that paramount lineage. Te Moanaroa had his senior line of descent through his mother, who was of a special rank awarded for skill- this shown by the double forehead rays on the right-hand side.* Original lithograph from two-volume set published in 1846 entitled *The New Zealanders Illustrated* by George French Angas.
**The Art of Maori Tattoo* by Dr. D. R. Simmons, published in 1986 by Reed Methuen publishers of Auckland, New Zealand.

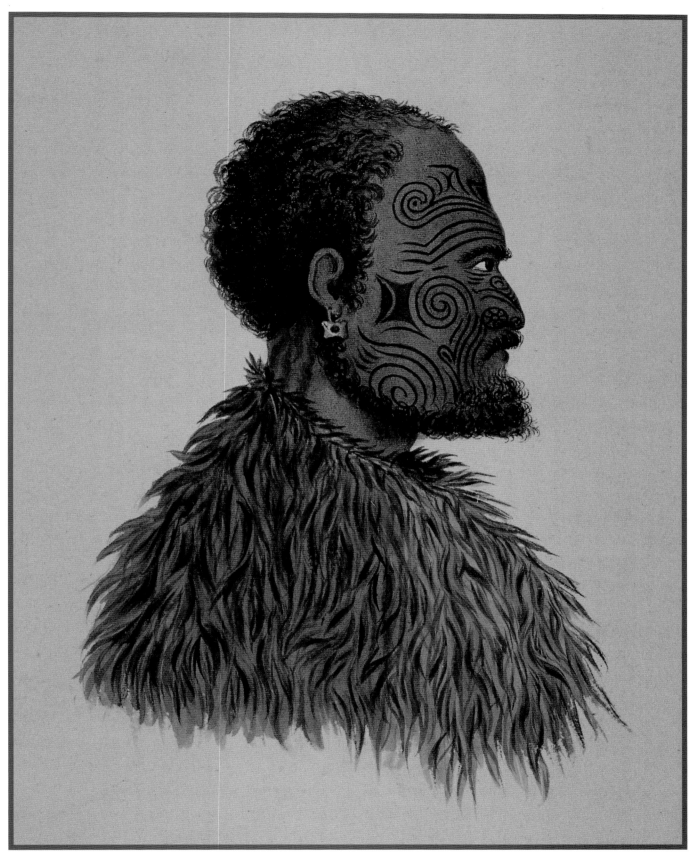

Original watercolor after John Savage* of "Tiarrah" of the Ngati Rehia of the Bay of Islands, North Island. It was John Savage who, in 1805, records tattoo as follows: "This society is divided into classes, each distinguished by devices variously tattooed on their faces and persons." According to Dr. D. R. Simmons in his book on Maori tattoo,** he describes this famous portrait: "At first sight his tattoo with forehead rays forming a spiral and the other figures on his forehead look very curious, but understandable. He is a man who was proclaimed a chief of a tribe descended from a paramount tribe. He has been granted these rights, which go to his descendants. The design by the ear is a particular mark of a paramount chief, Ruwaihou, whose protection is given."

*John Savage was a surgeon who traveled widely throughout New Zealand in 1805. His book *Some Account of New Zealand*, published in London in 1807, is considered a classic. This watercolor appears to be an early copy of his work.

**The Art of Maori Tattoo* published in 1986 by Reed Methuen publishers Auckland, New Zealand.

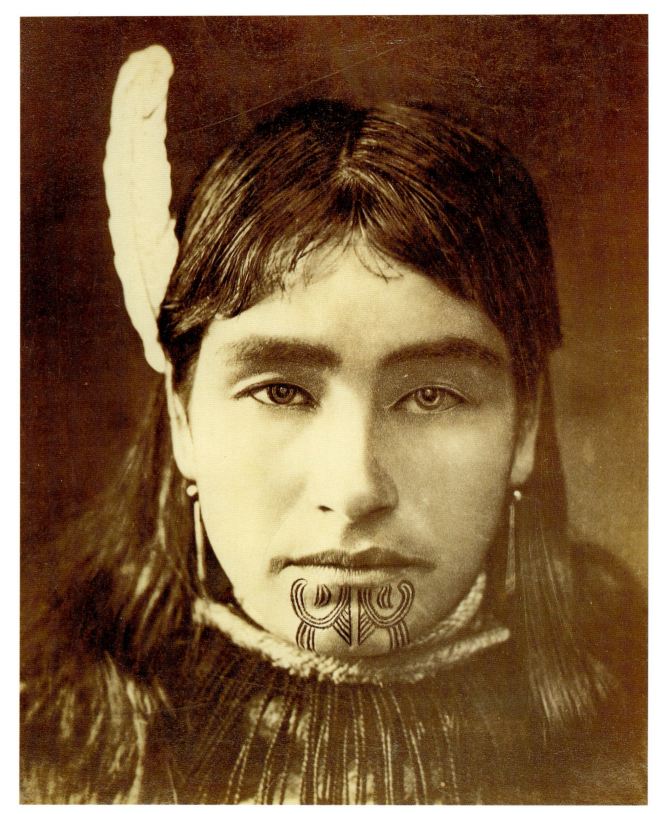

"Unknown Woman." An interesting portrait showing a chin tattoo that has been overly retouched by the photographer. Original albumen print mounted on board. Photographer unknown. Circa 1890s.

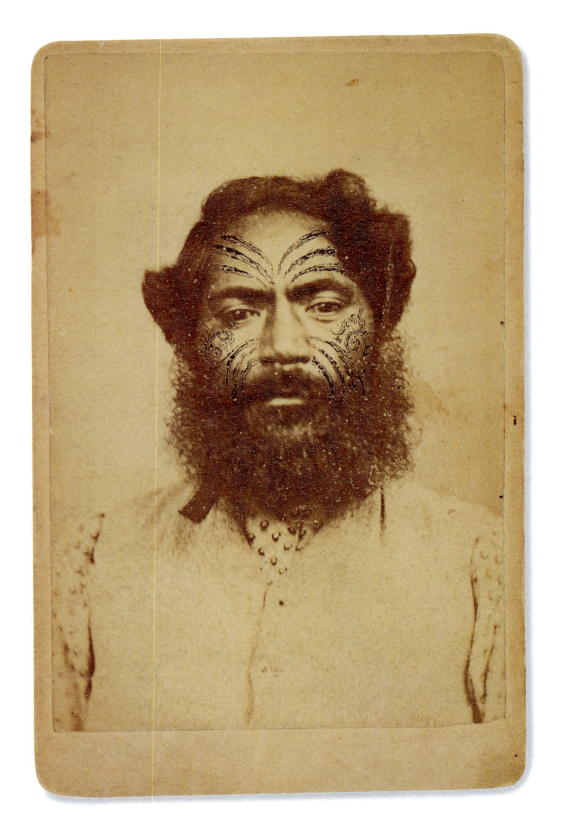

Carte de visite circa 1860s. A portrait of an unknown person. This image has been retouched by the photographer, enhancing the moko. Photographer unknown.

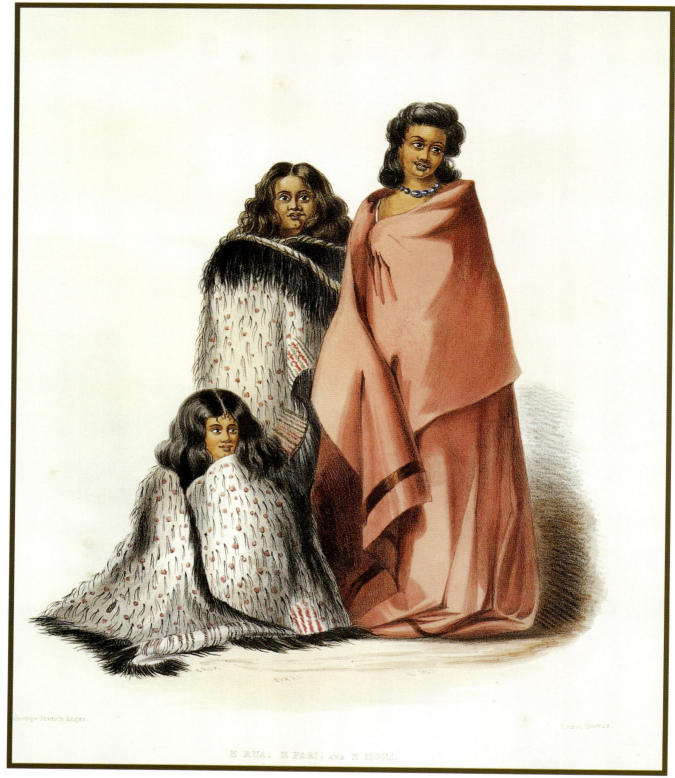

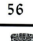

"E Rua, E Pari, and E Hoki." Drawn from life by George Angas, 1844. These three elegant ladies are of the Ngati Toa tribe residing at Porirua near Rangihaeatas *pa* on the shore of the Cook Straits, North Island. Two of the women shown here are adorned in traditional woven flax garments, while the third is wearing a red wool trade blanket so highly esteemed by the Maori people of this time period. The importance of this image is the lack of any tattoos on the women. Tattooing occasionally did occur on women prior to this time period, but did not come into wide fashion until after 1850. Original lithograph from two-volume set published in 1846 entitled *The New Zealanders Illustrated* by George French Angas.

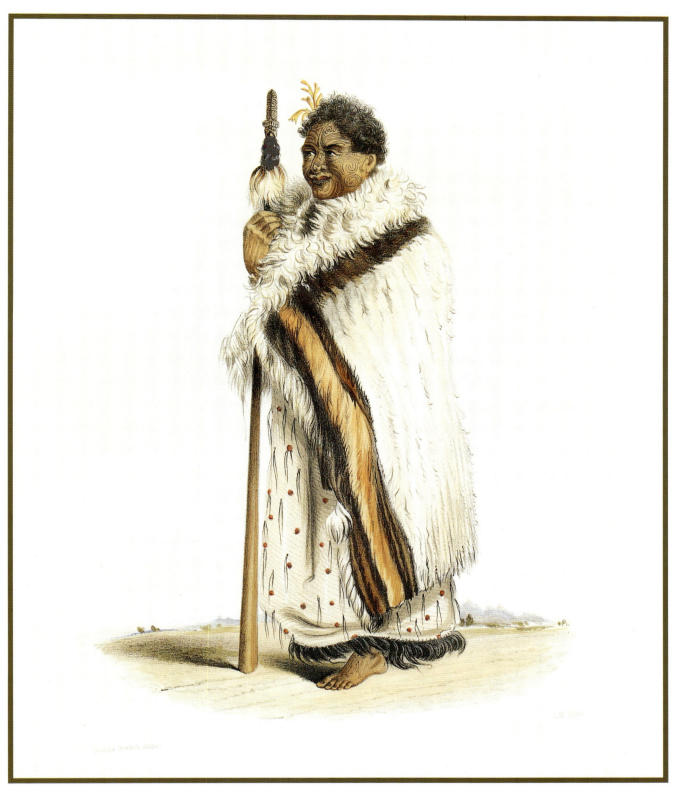

"Tamati Waka Nene." Drawn from life by George Angas, 1844. An important figure in New Zealand history as the first signer of the "Treaty of Waitangi." Being a chief of the Ngapuhi tribe, he was appointed by the United Tribes of New Zealand (Kohuiarau) as their spokesman at this historic signing. His central forehead moko design is that of a paramount chief. His father, Tapua was a *kohere*, a man of rank of Ngati Kahu lines, while Nene himself was of Ngapuhi and Ngati Kahu. He was an important figure throughout his life, dying in 1871. Original lithograph from two-volume set published in 1846 entitled *The New Zealanders Illustrated* by George French Angas.

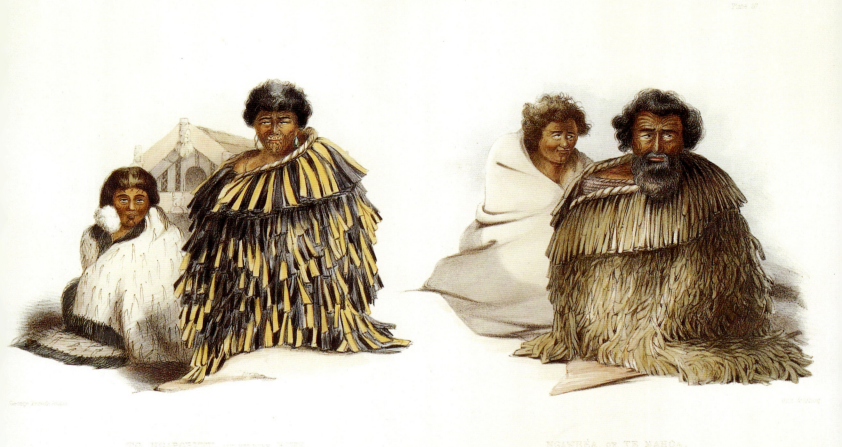

"To Ngaporutu and his wife Rihe at Wakatumutu – Ngawea, of Temahoa a chief of Ngatimaniapoto tribe, Nga Miho wife of Rangituaea." Drawn from life by George Angas, 1844. To Ngaporutu was chief of a small village in the district of Mokau, near Taupo in the North Island, the village name being Whakatumutumu. Known as a distinguished warrior and belonging to the Ngati Manipoto tribe, he embraced Christianity at the time of this drawing. His wife Rihe (with typical chin tattooing) was one of several wives he had taken. According to Angas, because of his recent conversion he had taken Rihe as his only wife. Angas also notes that Rihe was of the Wanganui tribe and had been purchased for thirty pigs. He further states that the cast-off wives were anxiously waiting for her to die, each one hoping that she was next in line. Nga Whea was one of the numerous chiefs of the Waikato tribe and was still practicing traditional Maori religious beliefs at the time of this drawing. Nga Miho (the teeth) was a celebrated "priestess," according to Angas, and was also one of the wives of Rangituataea. Angas was able to capture this pair in a dignified pose of great strength and wisdom. Original lithograph from two-volume set published in 1846 entitled *The New Zealanders Illustrated* By George French Angas.

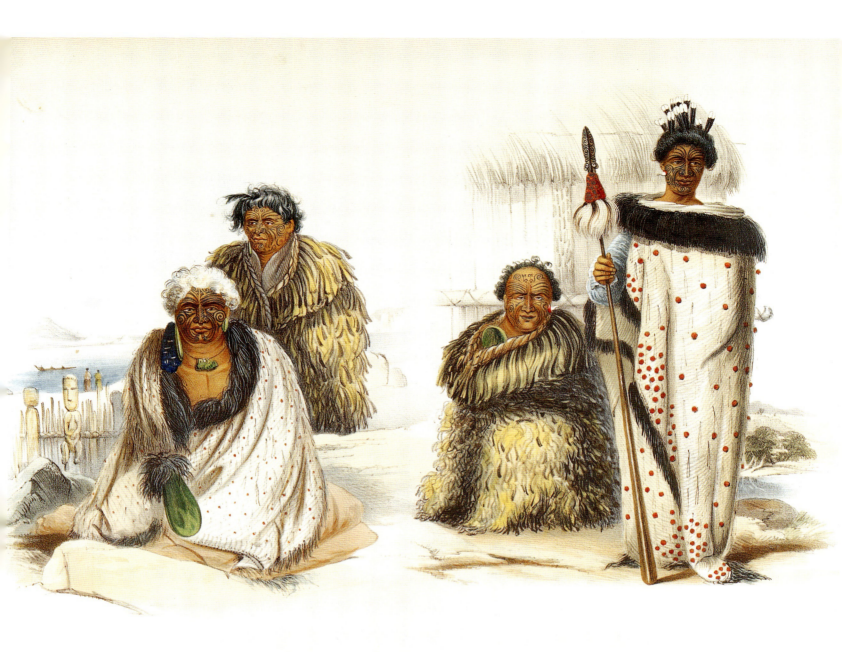

"Te Kawaw and his nephew, Te Heuheu, and Hiwikaw." Drawn from life by George Angas, 1844. Te Kawaw was the principal chief of the Ngat Whatua tribe near present-day Auckland. Among other things, he was famous for his large potato plantations. Here he is depicted with a jade *mere* in his hand and dressed in traditional flax garb with a tiger shark tooth earring. At his side is his nephew holding a *taiaha*, a weapon favored in combat, the lower end shown here at top with outstretched tongue motif. Te Heuheu Mananui or Tukino was principal chief of all of the Lake Taupo. He was by far the most important chief of the central North Island and was the *arikinui* of the Tuwharetoa tribe. According to Dr. D. R. Simmons, "The tattoo of Mananui has a forehead design in the center appropriate to a paramount chief of the second main line. Nose, upper cheek spirals and mouth rays also indicate male lineage on both sides."* Hiwikaw or Nga Papa was the brother of Te Heuheu. This was one of the last renderings of Te Heuheu, as he died shortly after this drawing in a landslide at Te Rapa. Original lithograph from two-volume set published in 1846 entitled *The New Zealanders Illustrated* by George French Angas.
The Art of Maori Tattoo by Dr. D. R. Simmons published in 1986 by Reed Methuen publishers of Auckland, New Zealand.

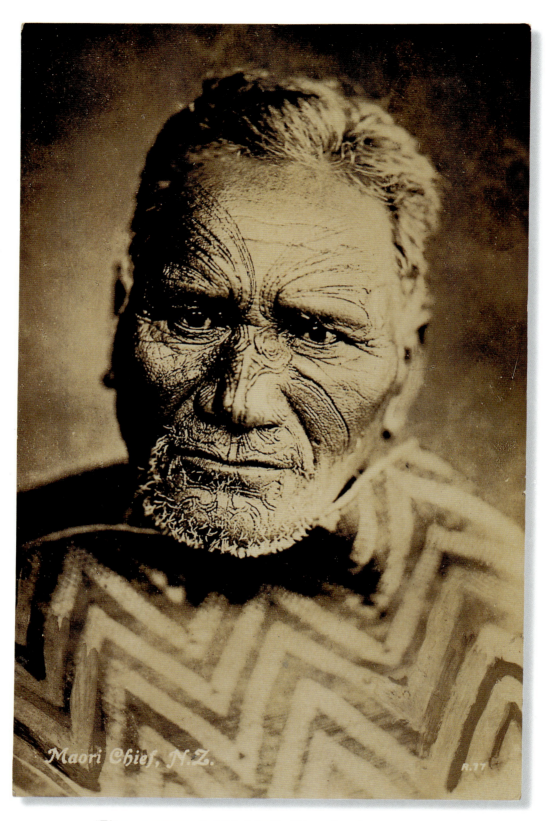

"Tihema a paramount chief of the Kai Tahu of the South Island." A portrait showing one of the South Islands more notable chiefs who lived at Kaikoura. A deep chisel moko applied clearly at the beginning of the 19th century, Tihema is shown in a reflective pose possibly contemplating the state of affairs that had come upon the Maori people. From original postcard entitled "Maori Chief, N.Z." Tanner Bros. Ltd. Maoriland Photographic series - Wellington, N.Z.

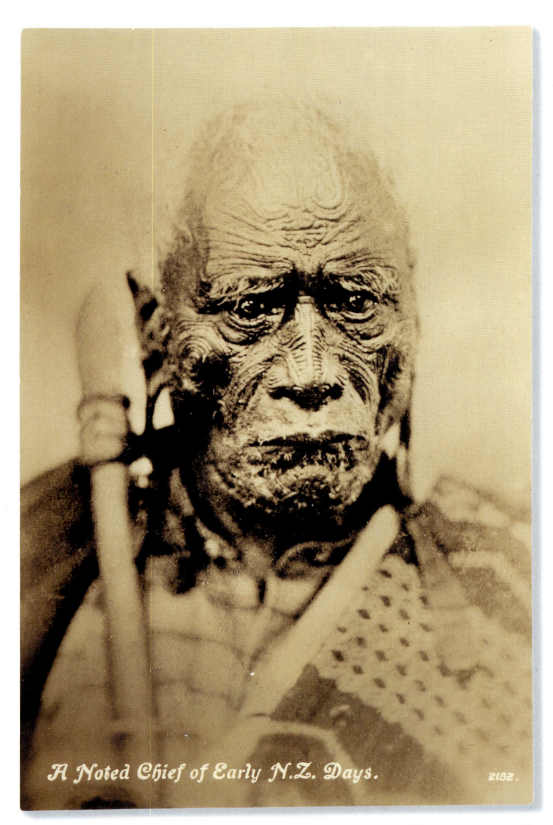

A Noted Chief of Early N.Z. Days.

"Taraia Ngakuti Te Tumuhuia." One of the most famous Maori chiefs exhibiting deep chisel moko. Leader of the Ngati tamatera tribe, he was often described in early New Zealand literature as being unscrupulous and treacherous, being one of the last to hold a "cannibal feast."* In 1830 he led a war party from the Upper Thames to Cook Strait where he joined the celebrated warrior Te Rauparaha and sailed with him to make war on the Ngaitahu at Kaiapoi in the South Island. From original postcard marked "A Noted Chief of Early N.Z. Days." Tanner Bros. Ltd. Maoriland Photographic series – Wellington, N.Z. circa 1910.

*In reality, he was responsible for many of the small bush wars around the district of Auckland during the early 19th century. He moved his people to the Bay of Plenty then moved back to Hauraki to get better trade with the Europeans, giving a local chief the right to cultivate his land but not build houses, which was a land claim. This local chief built houses, so Taraia descended on him, killed and ate him, thus absorbing the land claim. This was in 1844 after European settlement; hence he is often known as the "last of the cannibals," which he wasn't.

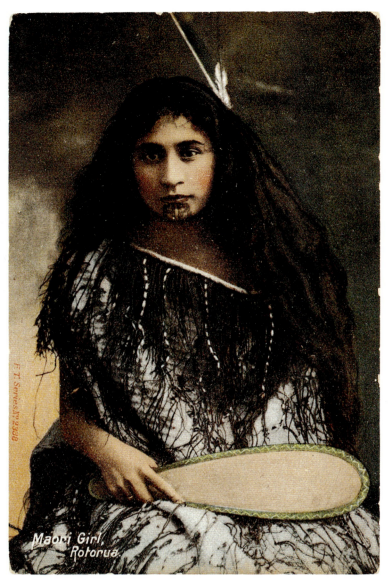

"Unknown Woman of Rotorua, North Island." In this photo, she is holding a whalebone ancestral club, *patu paraoa,* possibly indicating she is the oldest in the family. Her chin and lip moko is typical of the period and was done with the use of darning needles. From original postcard entitled "Maori Girl, Rotorua" F.T. Series #2338. Circa 1910/1915.

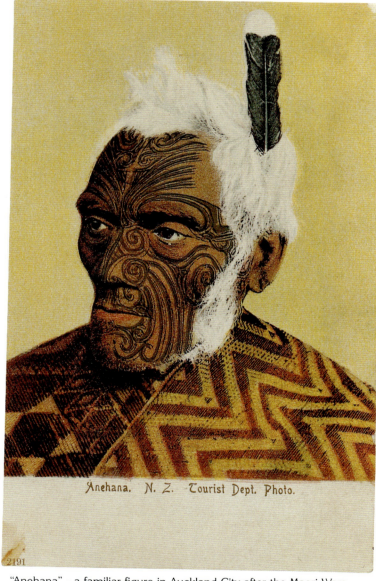

"Anehana" - a familiar figure in Auckland City after the Maori Wars. He was a favorite with early photographers and was painted numerous times by the artist Gottfried Lindauer. He was an excellent example of the old-time fully tattooed Maori rangatira. From original postcard marked F.T. series No. 2191 and labeled as a tourist department photo circa 1905.

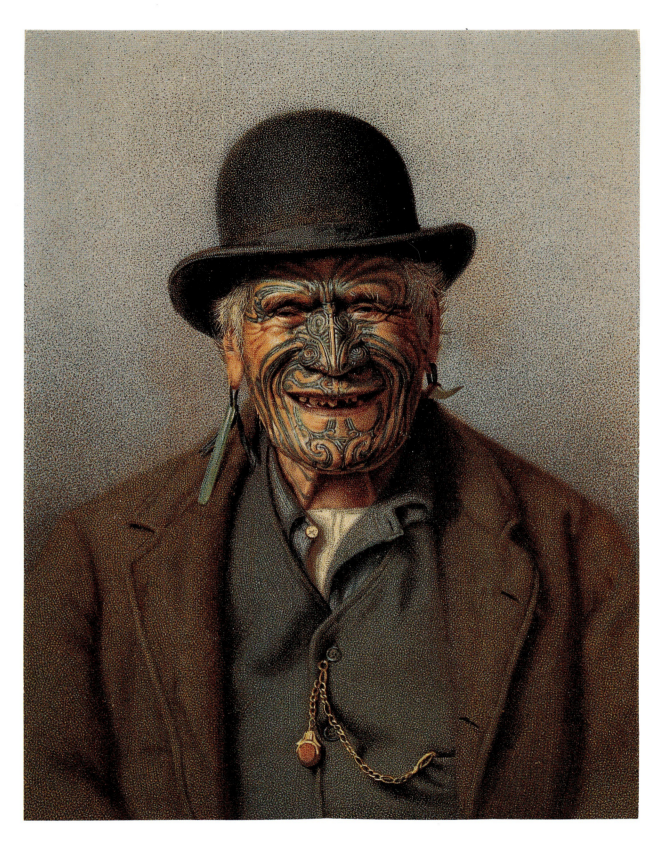

"A Good Joke ('Allee Same te Pakeha')." Te Aho te Rangi Wharepu, a chief of the Ngati Mahuta tribe of Waikato. This classic image is based upon a 1905 oil painting by noted New Zealand artist Charles Frederick Goldie (1870-1947) and was issued as a color lithographic postcard. In this image, Goldie emphasizes the moko that so fascinated the Europeans at this time. It is interesting to note at the peak of the postcard craze in 1909 between 9 and 14 million cards were posted in New Zealand.* Of this amount, it is estimated that over half depicted moko in some fashion. This image strengthens the stereotypical view so prevalent at this time period depicting the Maori people as 'happy go lucky,' lazy and not too bright. The danger was that views such as this were the only ones that many Europeans had at the time; this only strengthened the stereotypes of Maori people as inept and Europeans as culturally and racially superior. From original postcard circa 1905.

* For further information see *Delivering Views – Distant Cultures in Early Postcards*. Edited by Christraud M. Geary and Virginia-Lee Webb, Smithsonian Press, 1998.

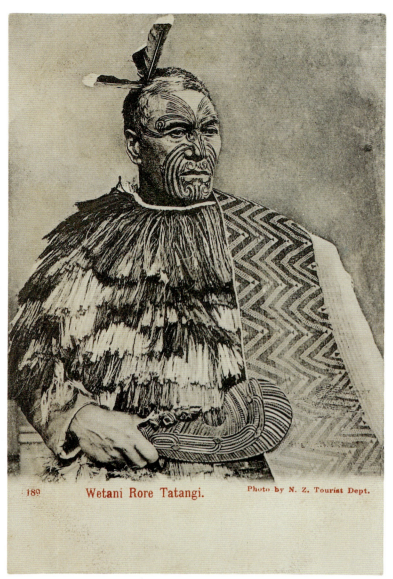

"Wetani Rore a chief of Ngati Maniapoto and Ngati Kahungunu, King Country." It has been suggested that the short lines on his forehead indicate that he was a teacher of weapons. An elegant studio portrait showing him wearing two types of flax cloaks and holding a late, ornately carved hand club known as a *wahaika*. From original postcard marked "Wetani Rore Tatangi," photo by N.Z. Tourist Dept. P.T. series no. 189 circa 1910.

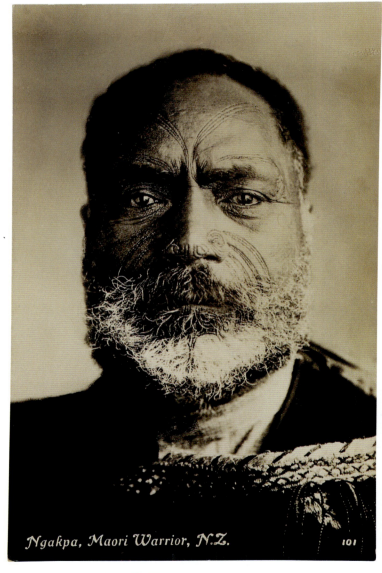

"Hori (George) Ngakapa Te Whanaunga of the Ngati Whanaunga, Ngati Paoa of Hauraki, North Island." A noted Maori warrior, he fought against the British in the Maori Wars near present-day Auckland. Much later he was a member of the Legislative Council (Senate) of the New Zealand Parliament. From original postcard entitled "Ngakpa, Maori Warrior, N.Z." Tanner Bros. Ltd. Photographic series – Printed in England circa 1910.

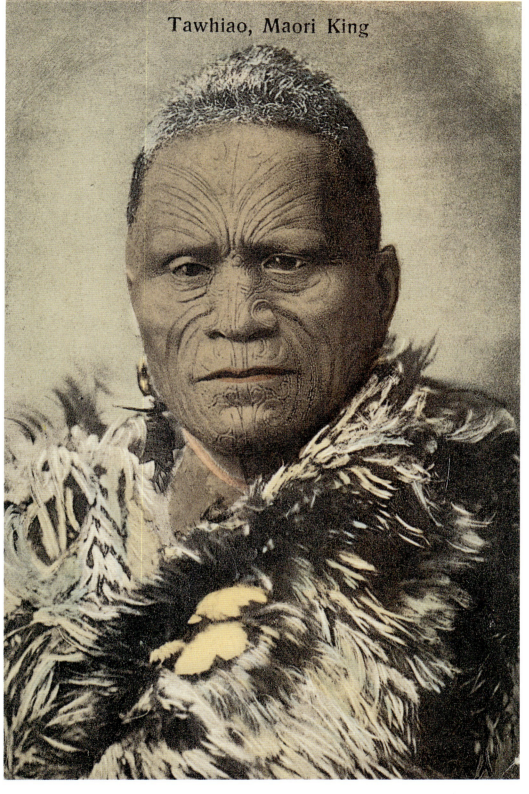

Tawhiao, Maori King

Tawhiao Potatau Wherowhero, also known as the Maori King. King Tawhiao was the son of Te Wherowhero, later known as Potatau, the first officially acknowledged Maori King. Tawahiao was declared King on his father's birthday in 1860. Of extremely high lineage, Tawhiao traced his ancestry to the chief who commanded the ancestral canoe *Tainui* during the migration from Hawaiki. This legendary chief Hoturoa plays an important part in Maori legend. Tawhiao was also connected by another line of descent with Tama te Kapua, the commander of the Arawa canoe in the migration from Hawaiki. Tawhiao was born in Orongokoekoe in about 1825. He was present at the battle of Rangiriri in 1863 and narrowly escaped with his life. After the Waikato war he retired into the King Country, isolating himself for over fifteen years. In 1884, he visited England with some other chiefs. Being a constant thorn in the side of the *pakeha* government, he was offered a pension in the year 1892, which he quickly returned on advice of the Maori council. The defiant return of this pension of two hundred ten pounds a year - a sizeable sum in those days - put his patriotism and integrity beyond doubt. The *Tangi* after his death was one of the largest in memory. From original postcard printed in Saxony and labeled W & A series circa 1905.

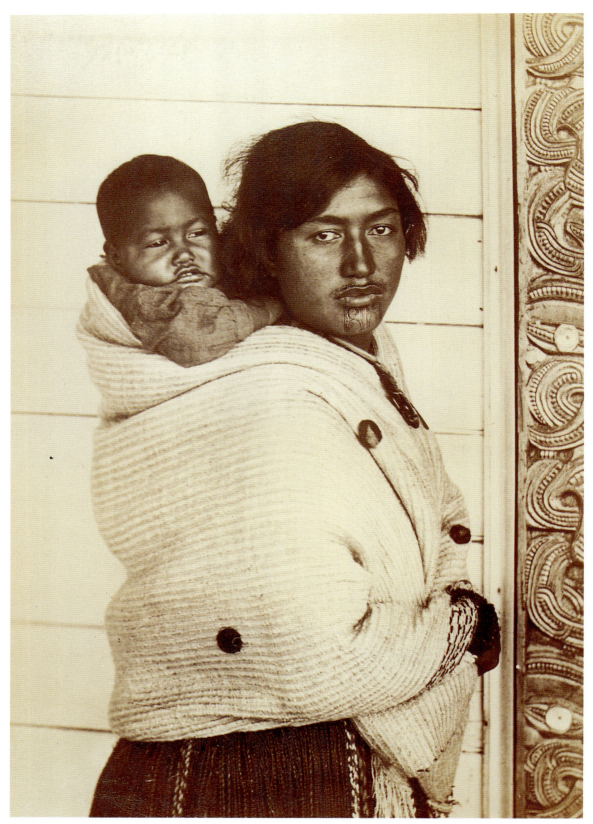

"Unknown Woman and Child." An image very popular with the tourists. This mother and child portrait is typical of the period. Original photograph mounted on board. Inscribed "Maori Pikau, Woman and Child, N.Z." 355 J.V. Circa 1890s.

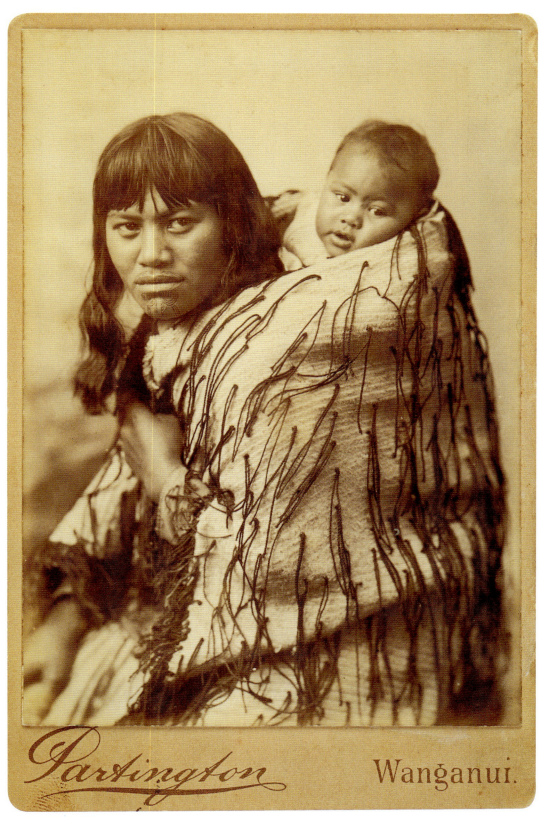

"Ana Rupene and Child." A woman of the Ngati Maru, Thames, Hauraki district of the North Island, she was often seen with a child on her back sauntering through the gold fields of the area. She was a favorite with photographers and was painted by Gottfried Lindauer around the turn of the century. Her portrait by Lindauer was universally admired and drew numerous tributes; when shown in St. Louis at the 1904 World's Fair, it garnered the exhibition's grand prize. A woman of great physical beauty, her moko, according to Dr. D. R. Simmons, shows descent lines on both sides. Original Cabinet Card marked under image: Partington, Wanganui.

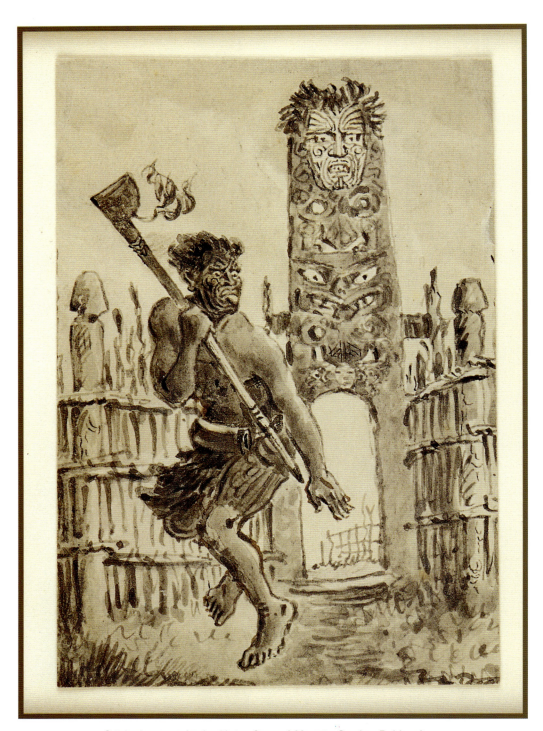

Original watercolor by Major General Horatio Gordon Robley. In this picture, the famous *pa* that stood at Te Ngae on Lake Rotorua is depicted with a Maori warrior in a defiant *haka* or war dance. In the warrior's hand is a *tewhatewha*, a type of war club, whose most striking feature is the straight edge behind the flat surface – the blade being used as a signaling device, the expanded surface making it clearly visible. Often, as in this picture, the lower side of the axe-like feature had a bundle of feathers attached to it that quivered in the wind adding to the drama. In this war dance, a constant thrusting out of the tongue and distortion of the blue lines of the moko formed a quivering network. One can only imagine the fear struck in the minds of the early European explorers and settlers upon meeting a group of Maori warriors in this pose. Circa 1860s.

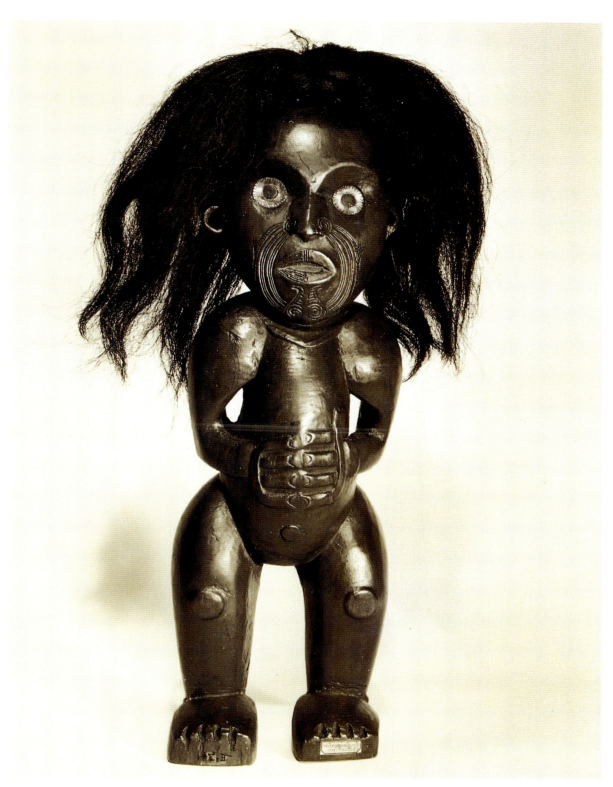

Free-standing image. This extremely rare male image with unusual moko is in the collection of the Hunterian Museum, University of Glasgow, Glasgow, Scotland. Clearly carved in the 18th century with stone or soft metal tools, this masterpiece is one of the few examples that exist.* It is generally thought that images of this type are closely related to other free-standing images in Polynesia and are religious in nature and function as abodes for the gods. Wood with paua shell eyes and human hair wig, 15-3/4 inches high. Original photograph taken by Dr. Terence Barrow in 1956.

*According to Barrow (1959) there are only five free-standing images in the world. In 1979 an additional one surfaced at Phillips Auction House in London realizing the sum of $146,000. This masterpiece is currently in the Dr. Murray Frum Collection in Canada.

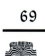

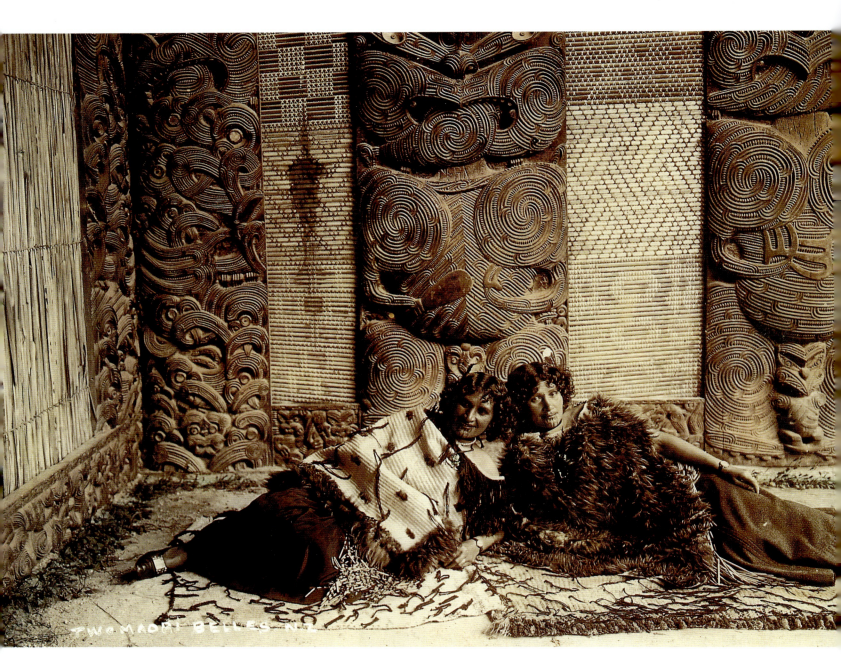

"Two Arawa Ladies in Maori meeting house." This lovely hand-colored photo was taken inside the Rangitihi meeting house. The house was carved in 1860 and stood at Maketu until 1897. This romantic and suggestive photo was published for the "tourist market" that was just beginning to fully emerge. These two unidentified ladies have traditional lip and chin moko, heightening their exotic appeal to the tourist market. Original mounted photo inscribed "Two Maori Belles" in white ink, photographer unknown.

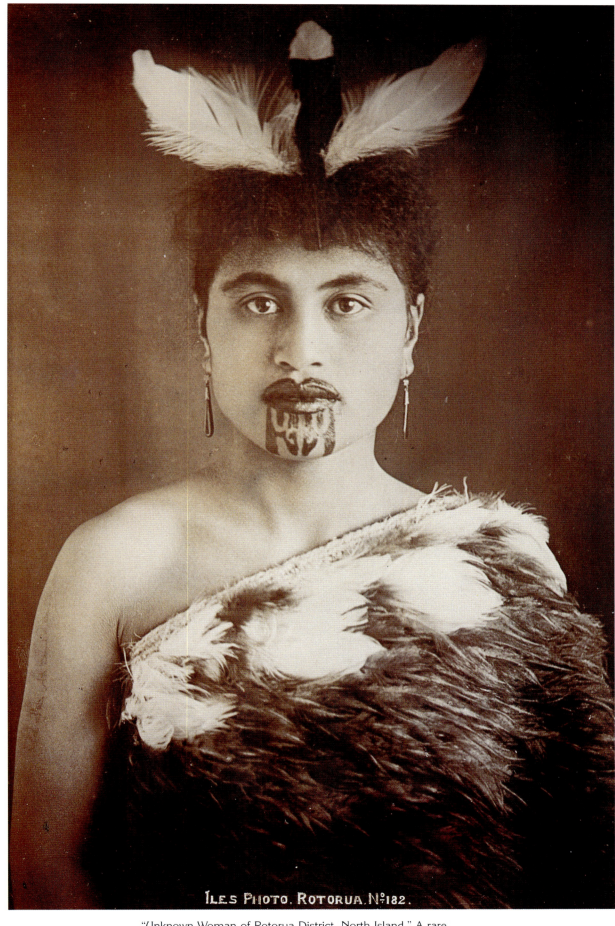

"Unknown Woman of Rotorua District, North Island." A rare portrait of moko applied by "grouped" darning needles around 1910 by tattoo artist Tame Poata. A wonderful photograph of this Arawa lady, undoubtedly of high rank. Original Albumen photograph by Iles. Circa 1910.

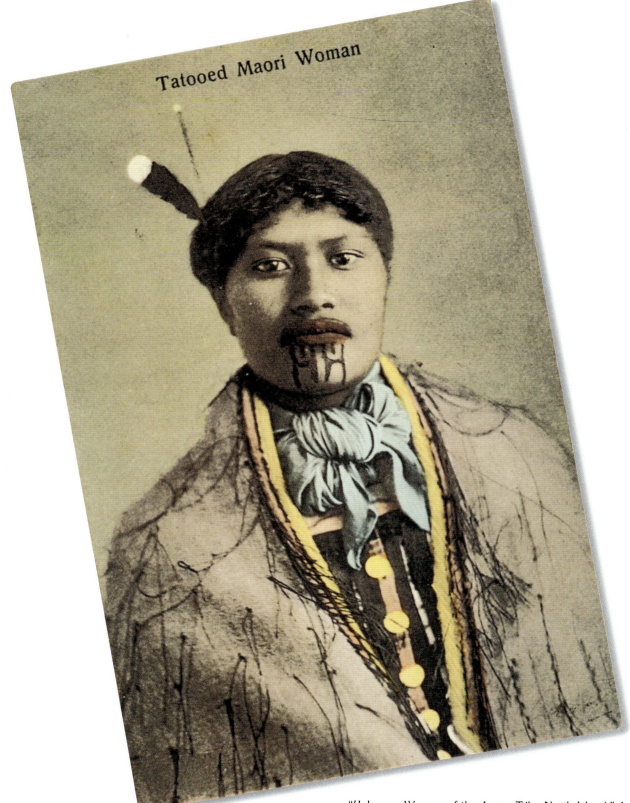

"Unknown Woman of the Arawa Tribe North Island." A rare image showing a tattoo done by Kahukuhu, a female tattoo artist, about 1910. This "grouped" darning needle tattoo represents one of the few images of the work of a known female tattoo artist. From original postcard entitled "Tattooed Maori Woman" W&A Series. Circa 1915.

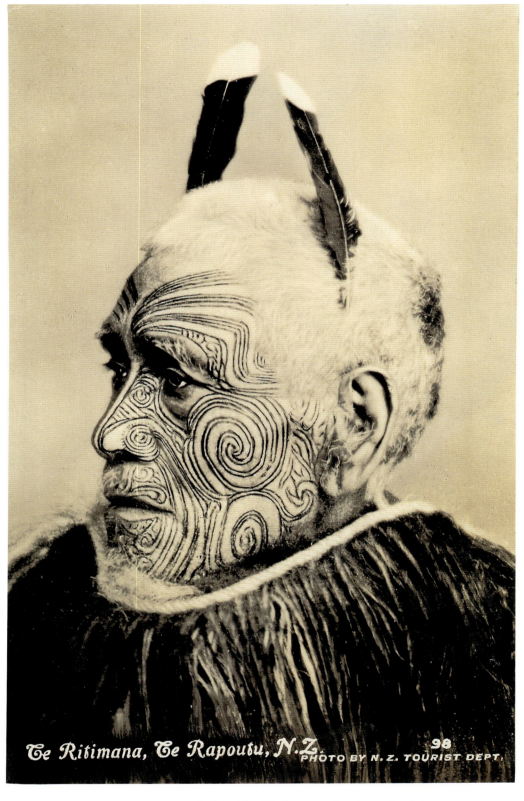

"Te Retimana a chief of the Ngai Tuwharetoa tribe situated at Lake Taupo, North Island." This heavily retouched photo shows the dignified chief with *huia* bird feathers in his hair. From original postcard entitled "Te Ritimana, Te Rapoutu, N.Z." Photo by N.Z. Tourist Dept. Tanner Bros. Ltd. Photographic series – Printed in England circa 1910.

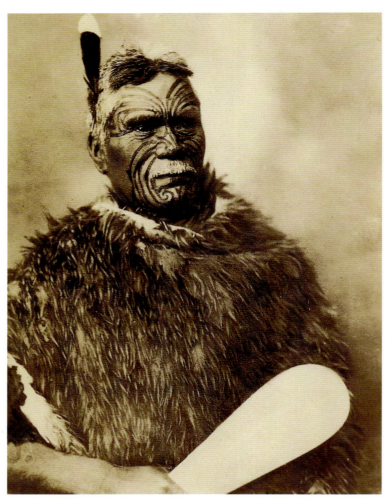
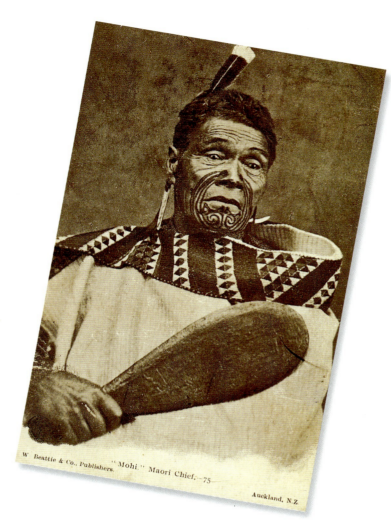

"Mahuta Te Toko, Ngati Maniapoto of the King Country and Ngati Kahungunu of Hawkes Bay, North Island." A minor chief of good standing but not a tribal chief in the true sense. In this photo he is shown in a traditional kiwi feather cloak, *kahu kiwi*, with whale-bone fighting club, *patu paraoa,* in his hand. This photo, like many of the period, shows an exaggerated moko with black paint or similar product used bringing out the ancient lines of this person who was quite elderly when this photograph was taken. A good example of early 19th century chisel tattoo work. From original real photo postcard simply marked on reverse "Post Card." Circa 1915.

"Mohi a Te Ngu, of Te Akitai, Ngati Mahuta of Mangere, Auckland North Island." A well-known personality around the environs of early Auckland. He often posed or dressed up for photographers without inhibitions. In this posed studio image he has a fine *kaitaka* cloak with wide *taniko* borders and a massive jade *mere* hand club in his hands. His pose, combined with the retouching done by the photographer, leaves the viewer with a disturbing, rather sad feeling. From original postcard entitled "Mohi Maori Chief #75" W. Beattie and Co. Publishers. Circa 1910.

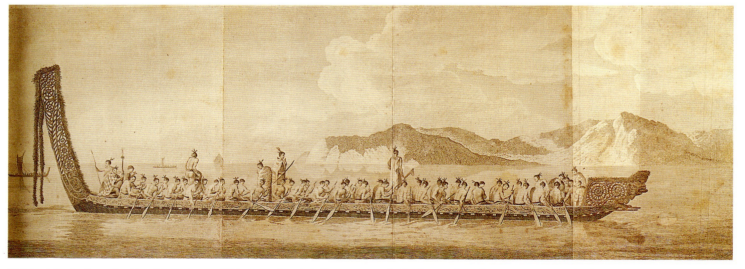

Original engraving of a Maori war canoe. This marvelous picture was drawn by Sydney Parkinson, artist with Captain Cook on his first voyage 1769-1770. The reason it is included in this book on tattoo is to show the reader that the classic spirals seen in facial moko can be found in canoe carvings as well as in various other art and artifacts of the Maori culture. This spiral is the most distinctive surface decoration in classic Maori carving. The use of spirals is closely paralleled in Borneo and New Guinea. In other areas of Polynesia, its closest parallel is in the Marquesas where the spirals tended to be rendered in a more rectilinear form. Circa 1784.

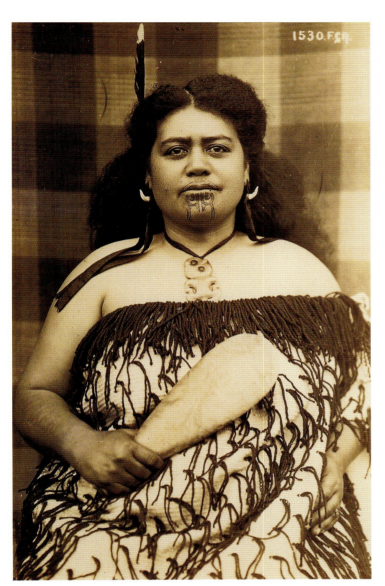

"Te Akau of Ngati Kahungunu of Hawkes Bay North Island." This powerful lady was also of the Ngati Toa of Porirua on the southwest coast near present-day Wellington. Related to the famous Te Rauparaha through her mother, Te Rangi Topeora, she succeeded her mother as commander of the tribal armies. It is interesting to note that she never had to fight or go to war. From original photo postcard marked on reverse "Frank Duncan & Co. Ltd." Circa 1920.

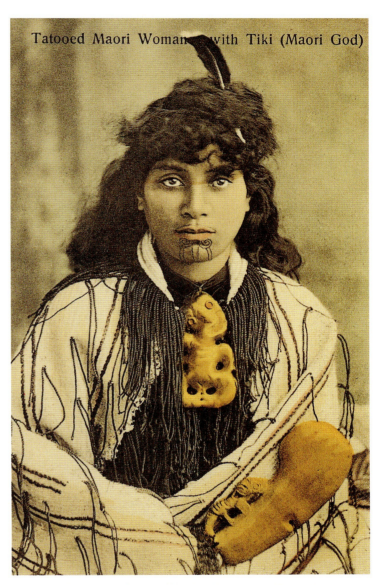

"Unknown Woman of Rotorua District, North Island." A typical tourist postcard aimed primarily at the visitors of the Thermal Springs District. In this photo all the exotic elements are present that were and still are a fascination to visitors: traditional clothing, *hei tiki*, *wahaika*, and, of course, moko. Original postcard entitled "Tatooed Maori Woman with Tiki (Maori God)." Reverse marked W&A Series. Phototyped in Saxony. Circa 1910.

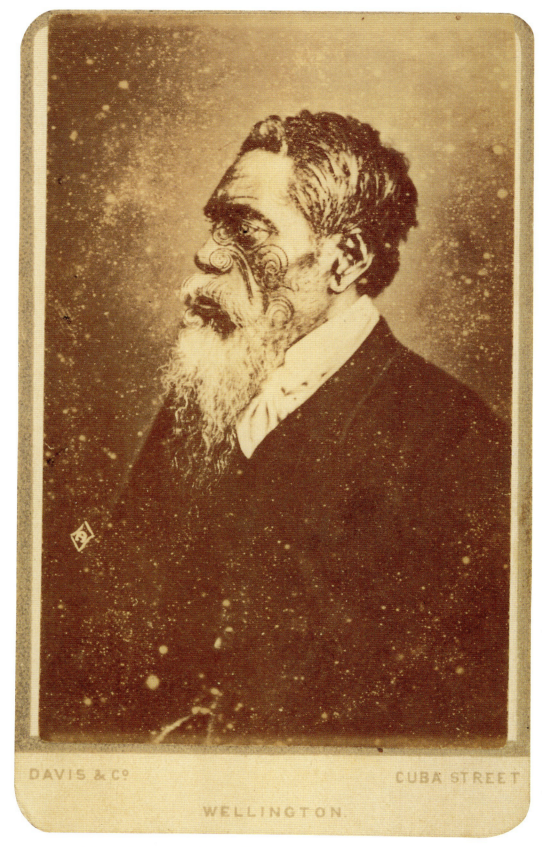

Carte de visite circa 1860s. A portrait of Renata (Leonard) Kawepo Tama ki Hikurangi of Ngati Upokoire, Ngati Kahungunu of Hawkes Bay, North Island. An important, well-known chief of high rank. He was one of the early lay readers with the Anglican Mission under the Rev. Colenso. He also was one of the more high-ranking chiefs to have fought with the Europeans and was in charge of the Maori Militia. On a more gruesome note, one of his eyes was gouged out by a woman during the fight against rebel leader "Te Kooti." Davis and Co. photographers, Cuba Street, Wellington.

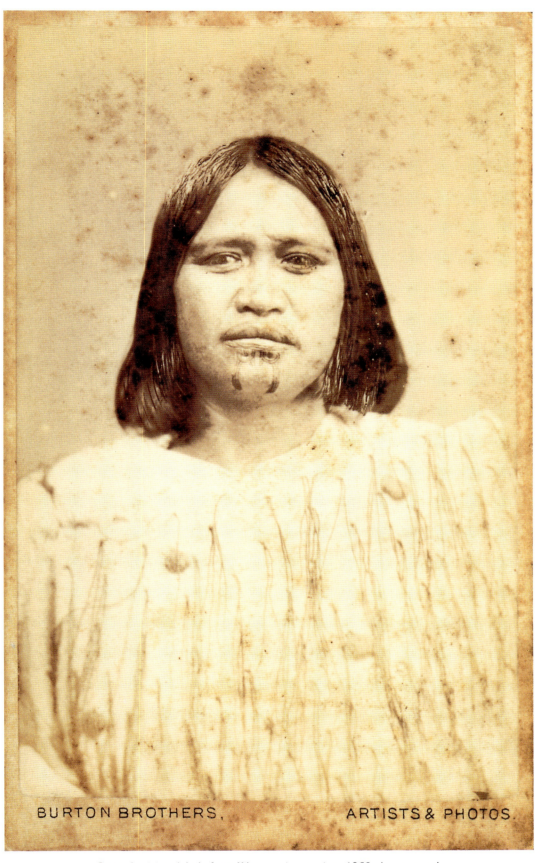

Carte de visite. A lady from Wanganui area circa 1860. A very good example of traditional women's tattooing done during the mid-19th century. Burton Brothers Photographers, Dunedin, N.Z.

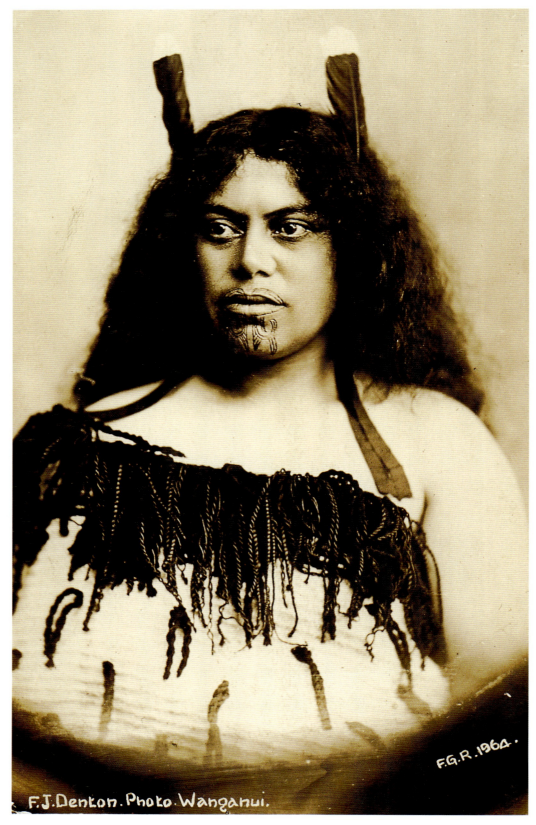

"Unknown Woman of the Te Ati Awa Tribe of Taranaki North Island." A lady from a family of rank, shown by her moko, according to Dr. D. R. Simmons.* This image portrays a different feeling than the usual female images of the time period. It has a more "wild, savage look" usually found only in male portraits. From original photo postcard marked at bottom "F.J. Denton Photo, Wanganui F.G.R. 1864." Circa 1915.
*Personal communication, 1998.

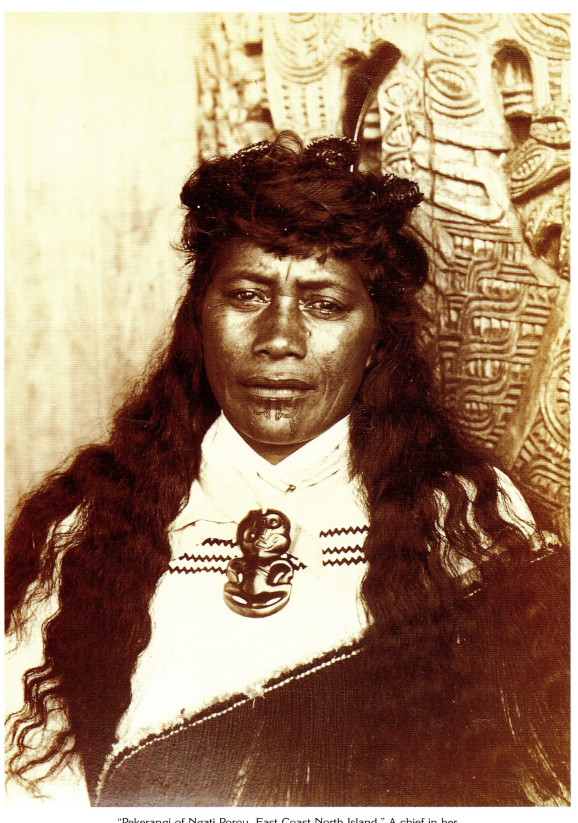

"Pekerangi of Ngati Porou, East Coast North Island." A chief in her own right, she could stand and speak on the *marae*, a place usually reserved only for men. In this powerful portrait, she is posed in front of a meeting house with a *hei tiki* around her neck. Original albumen photograph mounted on board entitled "Maori Wahine, Pekerangi. N.Z. 17363 J.V." Circa 1890s.

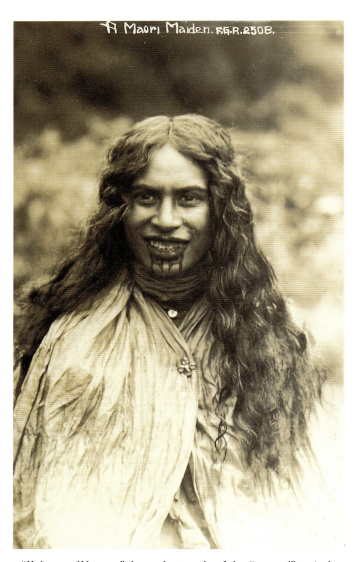

"Unknown Woman." A good example of the "second" revival in female tattooing around 1910 and done with the use of "grouped" darning needles. Original photo postcard entitled "Maori Maiden" F.G.R. #2508. Circa 1915/1925.

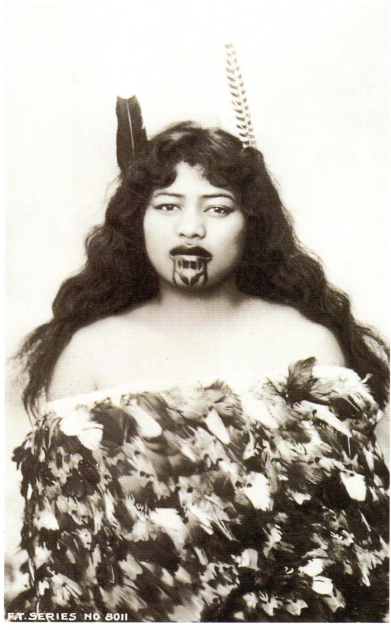

"Unknown Woman." Dressed in finery, including a pheasant feather cloak, she demonstrates both beauty and grace in this imposing photograph. Her chin and lip moko is typical of the period and was done with the use of "grouped" darning needles. From original photo postcard entitled "Maori Woman" F&T series #8011. Circa 1910.

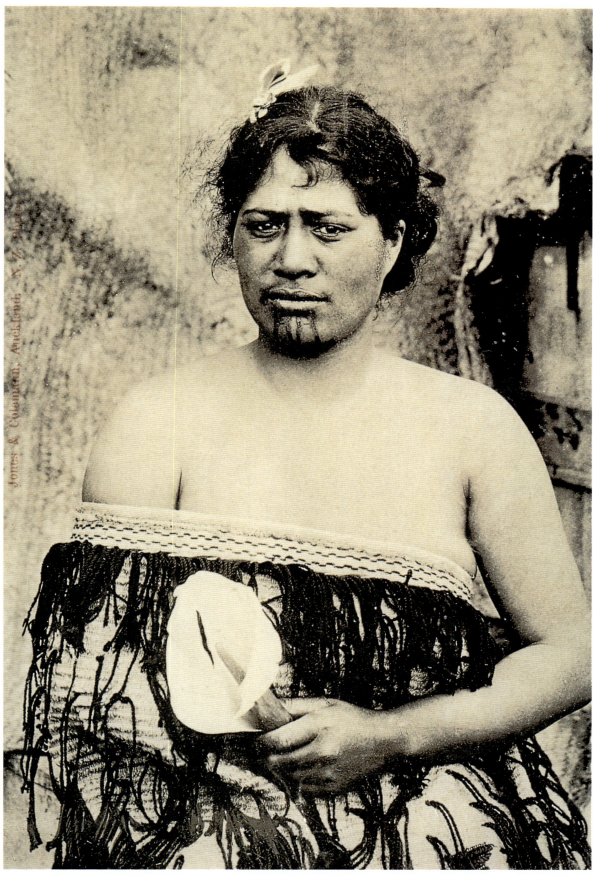

"Maori Lily (Rire)." Probably a lady from the Wanganui-Taranaki area of the North Island. A rather unusual use of the photographers imagination. From original postcard marked on reverse Joco Post Card – with Best Wishes and Compliments of the Season. Circa 1915/1920.

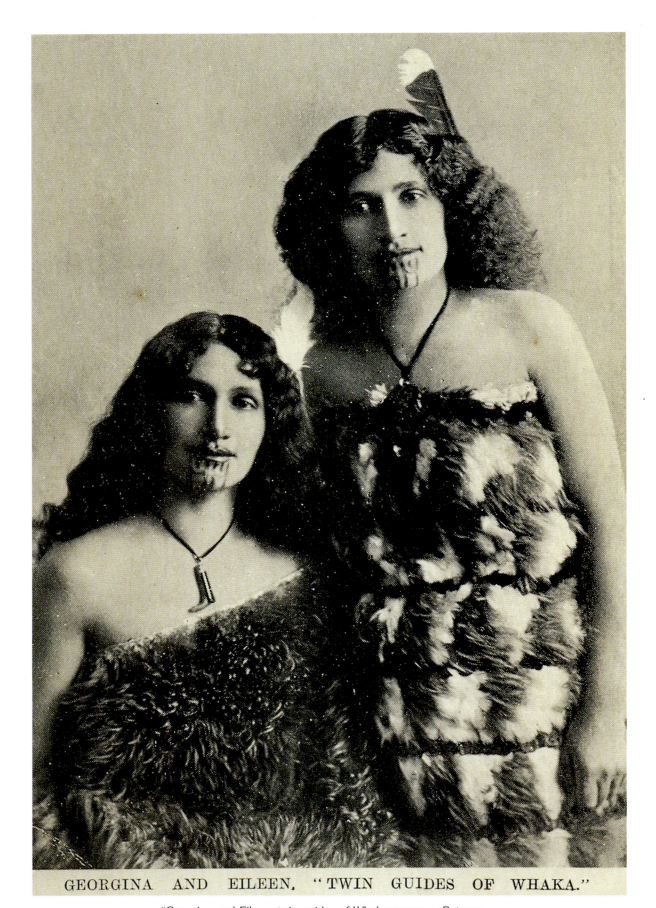

GEORGINA AND EILEEN, "TWIN GUIDES OF WHAKA."

"Georgina and Eileen, twin guides of Whakarewarewa, Rotorua North Island." These two Arawa sisters worked in the Thermal Springs District of Rotorua guiding early tourists around this famous area. A favorite with photographers and tourists, they are seen here both with chin and lip moko done with the use of darning needles. Original postcard by Iles circa 1910/1915.

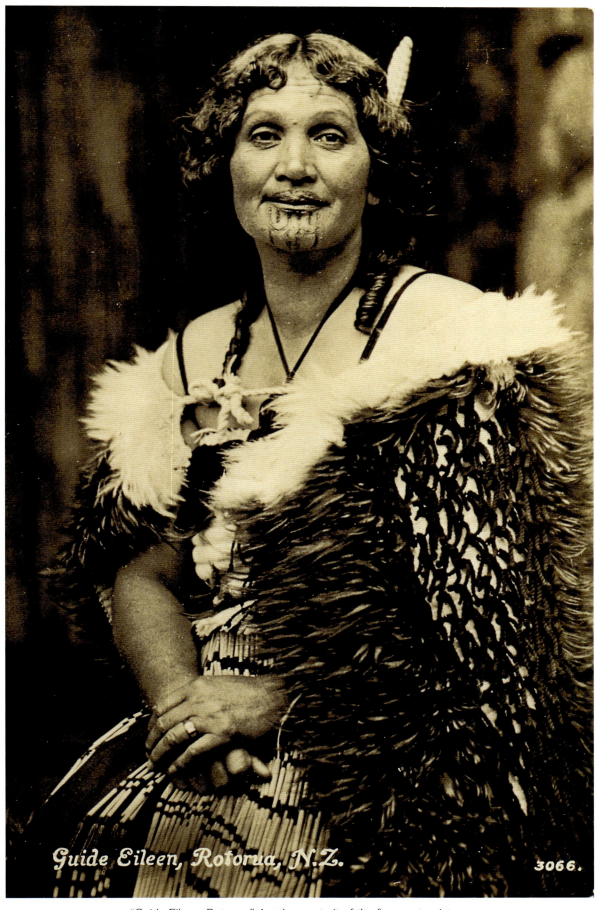

"Guide Eileen, Rotorua." Another portrait of the famous tourist guide, this time without her twin sister. From original photo postcard marked on reverse "Tanner Bros. Ltd. – Maoriland Photographic Series #3065." Circa 1915/1920.

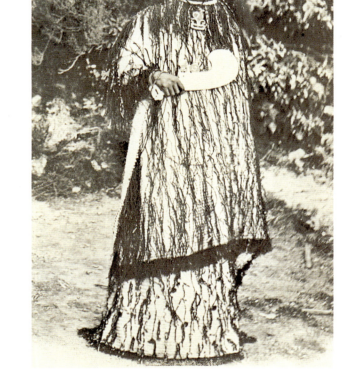

"Hikihiki of Nga Herehere of the Ngati Kahungunu tribe." An important woman in New Zealand history having a son, Aitu, by an English sea captain. Aitu was made a chief of the Queen Charlotte Sound area in the northern South Island. This photo originally taken in 1867* depicts Hikihiki in a flowing *korowai* dress cloak with whalebone hand club, *wahaika,* and neck pendant, *hei tiki,* around her neck. A chin and lip tattoo adds to her stately appearance. From original postcard entitled "A Maori Princess," #27 New Zealand Post Card. Circa 1905.
*Personal communication Dr. D. R. Simmons, 1998, for attribution and date.

Below: Artist rendering of the art of Maori tattooing. From original postcard printed by Ferguson and Hicks Wellington, New Zealand "Maori History Series #1" circa 1915. Caption on card reads as follows: "The Art of Mata-Ora – Tattooing the face of a Maori Chief (Moko). Tattooing was a favourite adornment of old-time warriors. In olden times a small sharp bone chisel was used to make the incisions, and a vegetable pigment was rubbed into the miniature trench in order to give the necessary blue coloring. With the men moko has long fallen into desuetude, but the native women of many of the tribes still have their lips and chins adorned with the modern tattooer's steel chisel."

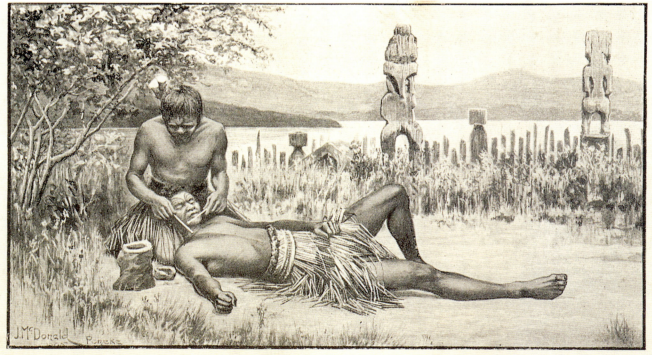

THE ART OF MATA-ORA—TATTOOING THE FACE OF A MAORI CHIEF (MOKO).

Tattooing was a favourite adornment of old-time warriors. In olden times a small sharp bone chisel was used to make the incisions, and a vegetable pigment was rubbed into the miniature trench in order to give the necessary blue colouring. With the men moko has long fallen into desuetude, but the native women of many of the tribes still have their lips and chins adorned with the modern tattooer's steel chisel.

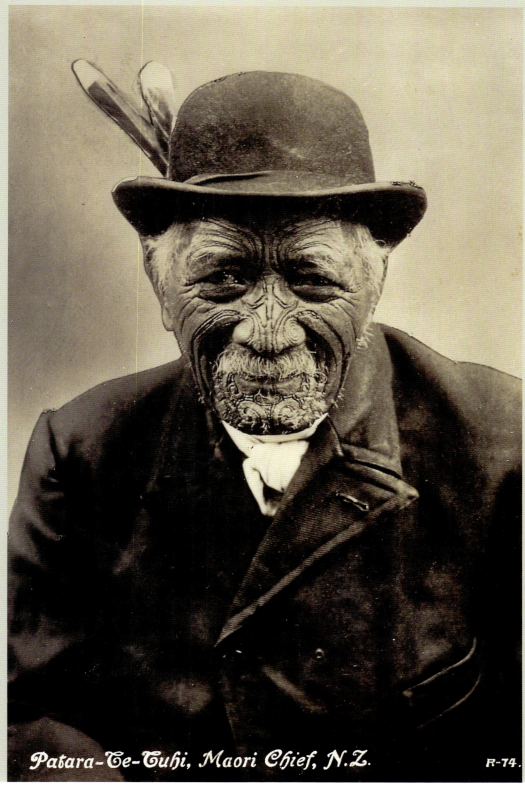

"Te Tuhi, Wiremu Patara chief of the Ngati Mahuta." One of the most interesting of the Waikato leaders, he attended mission schools in his youth and appears to have taken Wiremu Patara (William Butler) as his baptismal name. He was heavily involved in the "Maori King Movement" and became editor and principal writer of the newspaper *Te Hokioi e Rere Atu Na*, which became a pulpit for him in the interpretation of the Treaty of Waitangi. A noted warrior in the Maori Wars against the British at Waikato, he accompanied Tawhiao into isolation in the King Country for nearly 20 years. As the secretary for the Maori King Tawhiao, he handled negotiations with Premier Grey and in 1884 accompanied the King to England. At the turn of the century, he was one of the most admired men in New Zealand by both Maori and *pakeha* alike. He was well known for his shrewdness and good nature, dying in 1910. He was a favorite with photographers and artists. Charles F. Goldie painted him numerous times towards the end of his life. His moko is shown in a classic *waikato* style, although in Goldies' portraits he took artistic license to standardize patterns. In his lifetime, this notable Maori saw the coming of the *pakeha* and the near extinction of his own race. From original postcard entitled "Patara-Te-Tuhi, Maori Chief, N.Z.," Tanner Bros. Ltd. – Photographic series. Printed in England circa 1910.

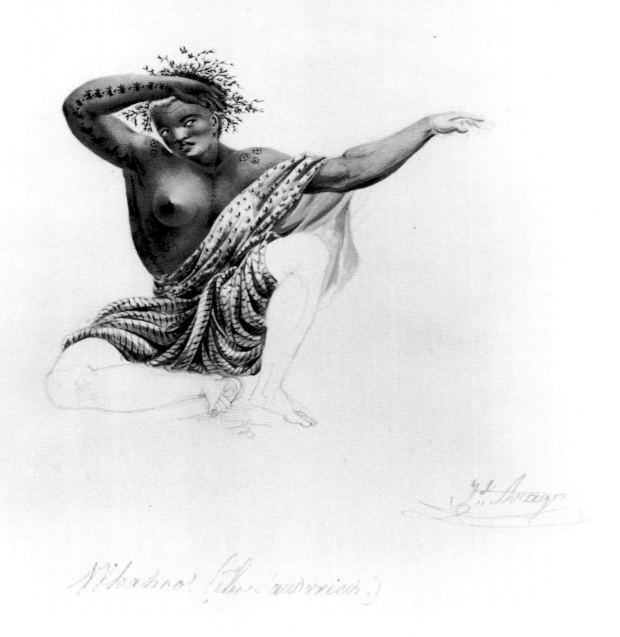

Original ink wash drawing by Jacques Arago entitled "Jeun Fille Dansan Wahoo" (Young Female Hula Dancer Oahu). In this superb uncompleted picture done in August 1819, a hula dancer is depicted with a row of goats going up her arm. On the opposite shoulder is a circle motif with inner cross design. *Honolulu Academy of Arts, Gift of Mark and Carolyn Blackburn.*

HAWAI`I

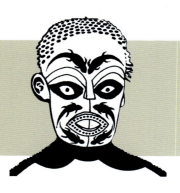

The Hawaiian Islands consist of eight primary islands -Niihau, Kaua`i, Oahu, Moloka`i, Lana`i, Maui, Kahoolawe, and Hawai`i. Considered to be one of the most isolated groups of islands on earth, they are located over 4,000 miles from New Zealand and 2,000 miles from the coast of California. These "high islands" are volcanic in origin and rise to over 13,000 feet on the island of Hawai`i at the summits of Mauna Kea and Mauna Loa. The terrain remains varied from island to island, with the windward areas tending to be cool and moist, and the leeward, warm and dry. On the island of Hawai`i alone there is a 7- to 200-inch variation in rainfall and is representational of most of the islands. Erosion of the lava rock has provided fertile soil in areas of high rainfall, allowing for a rich harvest of agricultural goods; this soil is especially good for the cultivation of *taro*, which when pounded is known as *poi*, a mainstay in the ancient Hawaiian's diet. Forests once covered large areas of land, but these are now greatly depleted on all the islands due to clearing off for sugarcane and pineapple plantations and development, in general. Today the majority of the population resides on the island of Oahu, although in ancient times the island of Hawai`i was the most inhabited. Tourism is the main source of the economy today, and the islands are often referred to as the Paradise of the Pacific.

There are many schools of thought on the origins of the Hawaiian people. It is generally believed that the first migration originated from the Marquesas Islands around 600 AD, and a second migration from Tahiti at a later date.[1] The earliest of these voyagers came well equipped for settling by bringing with them various food plants and mammals such as dogs, fowls, and pigs.[2] During the period up to European contact the population grew and tribal territories were established under hereditary rulers.

Captain Cook is credited for being the first non-Polynesian to sight the islands, but in reality the Spanish - as far back as 1527 - may have sighted or made contact with the islands. Also the odd Japanese fisherman may have strayed off course, but these all remain unproven possibilities. There is no doubt that Cook was the first to have any extensive communication even though the Hawaiians already had small quantities of iron (*hao*) in their possession. Cook first viewed the island of Oahu in January 1778 and sailed past and anchored off Kaua`i. His first encounter with the Hawaiians was a friendly one, and he encountered a surprising reverence. After provisions were procured he briefly visited Niihau where some trading of curiosities of native manufacture occurred. It was on Kaua`i, though, that he records the first observation of Hawaiian tattooing:

> Tattowing or staining of the skin is practised here, but not in a high degree, nor does it appear to be directed by any particular mode but rather by fancy. The figures were straight lines, Stars & ca and many had the figure of Taame[3] or breast plate of Otahiete, though we saw it not among them.

To honor his patron the Earl of Sandwich, the first Lord of the Admiralty, he named the group the Sandwich Islands. Cook then proceeded north, the purpose of the voyage to search for a northwest passage to the North Atlantic.

At this time, Hawaiian society was stratified according to rank, being dependent on an individual's descent. The purest and most important one containing revered ancestors, who were held to be themselves descendants of gods. Descent was reckoned in both lines, and if a chief married a woman of lower rank, his children's standing would be proportionately lower than his own.

The highest rank was that of *ali`i*, and the senior male with the highest pedigree the chief or *moi*. Such hereditary rights were not always secure from challenges of high-ranking kin, and the widespread custom of adoption so prevalent through all Polynesian society made the genealogical situation extremely complex.

One of the most unusual aspects of Hawaiian society was the *kahunas* or "experts." Not necessarily of high birth, they operated in both religious as well as secular fields. These *kahunas* had skills in many areas including priestly ritual, house building, canoe construction and image carving. The majority of the population, though, were commoners or *maka'ainana* who occupied the land at the want and pleasure of the district chiefs. These people supplied the chiefs with tribute in the form of foodstuffs, *kapa*,[4] and other goods. Most of the items collected then would be given to the senior chief who would use these items in feasts and sacrifices, which were such a integral part of religious observances in ancient Hawaii. Another small portion of society at this time was the *kauwa* class. Greatly despised, this group was made up of prisoners and social outcasts and performed the most menial of tasks.

Engraving depicting a Hawaiian woman. This print, published in the 1820s, shows a rather fanciful depiction of a woman wearing tattoos. Published in Germany.

As in all Polynesia, society was held in check by a strict *mana* and *kapu* (taboo) system of religious beliefs. One of the more severe aspects of this was the penalty of death for a commoner's failure to prostrate himself in front of a chief; even his shadow falling on a chief would mean instant death.

Religious observances were centered on the *heiau* or sacred compound. In this area, elaborate rituals were performed by the priestly *kahunas*. These could last for several days and involved human sacrifice although cannibalism was not practiced as in New Zealand and Fiji. The principal gods were those recognized throughout Polynesia. These included Ku *(Tu)*, Kane *(Tane)*, Lono *(Rongo)* and Kanaloa *(Tangaroa)*. There were numerous versions of these major deities and many were patrons of daily activities. It was the god Lono, in fact, that Captain Cook was mistaken for by the Hawaiians. The god Lono was the god of peace and agriculture, and it is thought that because the ships' masts and sails appeared similar to the emblem of the god, Cook was seen as a reincarnation of Lono. This was one of the most unfortunate situations to have occurred in the annals of Pacific history. Wearing out his welcome on his first visit to Kealakekua Bay during the annual *makahiki* celebrations, he returned there due to a broken mast and later was killed in a skirmish at Ka'awaloa on February 14, 1779. In fact it has been suggested that it was the Hawaiians' disbelief in how the god Lono got himself into such a predicament as simple as a broken mast that contributed to Cook's problems upon his return and his ultimate death.

Representations of the gods were usually in human form and were constructed of various materials including wood, stone and basketry, although, as in most areas of Polynesia, pieces of unworked stone were sometimes subject to great veneration.

Hawaiian culture greatly changed with the arrival of the Europeans. Having had enough of the burdensome taboos that foreigners violated with apparently no effect, the chiefs and priests were ready to urge abolition of the *kapu* system. The opportunity to do this came when Kamehameha I died on May 8, 1819. This symbolic event occurred when Kamehameha II, urged by his two most powerful female chiefs, dined publicly at a table prepared for females in open violation of one of the most fundamental taboos of free eating or *'ai noa*. Thus, in this one dramatic gesture, the entire structure of the ancient religion collapsed.

In an unusual fate of timing, fourteen missionaries arrived on the brig *Thaddeus* six months later, totally unaware of the events that had just taken place. Having just discarded their traditional religion, the Hawaiians were eager to adopt this new Calvinist-based form of Christianity. Over the next 28 years, the American Board of Commissions for Foreign Missions, based in New England, was responsible for sending 12 companies totaling 140 men and women to the islands, many bringing their families. This event, along with the discovery of the islands by Cook in 1778, was one of the single-most important events, changing the islands forever.

In the years that followed there was an influx of trading activities as the islands became a center for whaling and the like. Following this, many of the missionaries became powerful business leaders with vast tracts of real estate. These were strengthened with powerful alliances with Hawaiian nobility through marriages or other compacts. Sugarcane then became king with vast plantations on all the major islands. It was, in fact, the revenue from this new source of wealth that allowed the last reigning king of Hawai`i, David Kalakaua, to travel around the world and build an ornate palace in the 1880s. Upon his death in 1891, his sister, Queen Lili`uokalani, took over the throne only to be ousted by a group of American businessmen in 1893. It was only a matter of time until the United States annexed the Hawaiian Islands in 1898, with ensuing statehood officially granted in 1959.

Today the island paradise is suffering with a severe case of economic malaise. Years of unbridled speculation by Asian interests in the 1980s and the islands' lack of diversification subsequently has caused turmoil and despair, especially in the native Hawaiian community. Gone is agriculture, with virtually all the plantations shut down, leaving many in the native community without work. Because of these economic and related factors, a renaissance has taken place with the call for Hawaiian sovereignty. In 1993 the United States officially apologized for the overthrow of the Queen, but this is hardly sufficient, and only time will prove what course the native Hawaiian people choose for their own destiny.

Hawaiian Tattooing – *kakau*

The Hawaiian technique of tattooing was similar to most other areas of Polynesia. It consisted of pricking the skin with a toothed tattooing comb carrying a dark vegetal pigment. Once the dye was under the skin it would remain in a permanent state, creating deep blue or black markings in a variety of forms.

In Hawai`i the process of tattooing may have been more guarded than in other areas of Polynesia. Being *kapu,* the process appears to have been very secretive, at least to Westerners' eyes. William Ellis, Captain Cook's surgeon, was the first person to attest to this by his following account:

> We never saw the operation of tattooing performed, nor could we procure a sight of the instruments used upon this occasion.

Tattooing was always a very painful and time-consuming process. The needle was made of the bone of the albatross, hence the name *moli*, which when translated[5] is the word for Laysan albatross. There is speculation as to the name of the mallet, with most scholars accepting *ku'au*, which when translated literally means "a mallet used for beating." There are very few examples of these instruments in existence today, possibly because of the sacredness and volatility of blood. After each use these items were probably destroyed; in fact, most needles known to have survived are from archaeological midden deposits and seem to support this theory.

In most instances, pigments used in the tattoo ink were derived from the soot and remains of the burnt kukui nut. This nut, often referred to as the candlenut, was found throughout the islands of Polynesia and had a variety of uses in ancient Hawai`i, including as a source of lighting, medicine and dye. The gum from this nut was also used in assorted activities including bird catching.[6] In 1819, the artist Jacques Arago[7] recorded that the kukui nut soot was mixed with the juices of the coconut and sugarcane, undoubtedly to thicken the mixture so the color would not run when entering the skin, thus assuring a clear crisp design. His description of the tattoo process is one of the few accounts recorded and appears to be most accurate:

> They fix the bone of some bird to a stick, slit the bone in the middle, so as to give it two or three points, which they dip in black colour... they apply these points to the part to be tattooed, and then they strike gently on the stick to which the bone is attatched, with a wand, two feet in length.

Who was tattooed in ancient Hawai`i and for what reasons appears to be a complex matter. Dr. Adrienne Kaeppler, noted scholar from the Smithsonian Institution in Washington, DC, has stated her hypotheses as follows:[8]

> ...that like other Hawaiian art forms, tattoo was a visual manifestation of social relationships among the people, the gods, and the universe that changed over time; that tattoo was primarily a protective device and a function of genealogy; and that the evaluative ways of thinking about tattoo (aesthetics) can be related to ways of thinking about other Hawaiian art motifs, processes, and an important aesthetic concept dealing with veiled or layered meaning known in Hawaiian as kaona.

This certainly appears to be the strongest argument put forward, but only the ancient Hawaiians have the true secret.

The concept of the tattoo as a protective device seems to come through other areas of Polynesia as well, especially the Marquesas where the full body tattoo acted as a type of armor. In fact, it was probably the function of male tattoo prior to the adoption of European weaponry that guarded the warrior, especially those of high rank. The actual process of tattooing combined with chants done at the time enveloped the wearer with a type of permanent sacred protection. This male tattoo was placed in several areas of the body including the legs, arms, torso and face. Memorial tattoos were also recorded from Cook's voyages onward. It was Arago who, for the first time, sketched the memorial tattoos of Kamehameha who had just died prior to his visit in 1819.[9]

Women were also tattooed, with the majority of the tattoo work done on the fingers, hands, tongues and wrists. There is much debate as to why women were tattooed, but it appears to be genealogically and spiritually

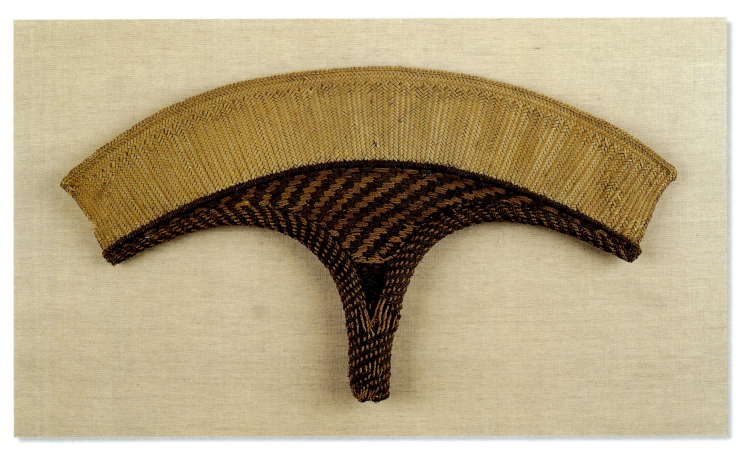

Hawaiian crescent fan or *Peahi niu*. This rare example is one of the few fans known to have survived. Woven of plaited pandanus interwoven with human hair. This art form surpasses anything in design and form in Polynesia and represents the highest achievement in the basketry arts. Reserved for people of high rank only, the crescent fan motif is encountered in traditional Hawaiian tattoo design. Width: 15 inches. 18th century.

based. It is a generally accepted fact that women in Polynesian society attract *kapu* and that they were closer to the gods; whether this has any relationship to tattooing remains to be seen. Some tattooing may have been purely decorative with no genealogical or spiritual meaning whatsoever; this certainly appears to be the case at the beginning of the 19th century when a variety of new designs appear in tattoo.

Tattoos seen by the first European explorers primarily consisted of linear motifs with rows of triangles, crescents, arches and chevrons. Lizards motifs or *mo'o* were also recorded. Captain Cook was the first to report such a design on the island of Niihau. The lizard held a special sacred place throughout Polynesia and was greatly respected and even feared.

The zigzag design made up of triangle and chevron elements, Dr. Kaeppler has argued, is symbolic of the backbone and genealogical concepts. She further states the crescent arches, or *hoaka,* are the same designs found on Hawaiian drums (*pahu*) and may be "symbolic of human beings joined together as lineal and collateral descendants who trace their relationships back to the gods."

Other important early references to tattoo include David Samwell, of Captain Cook's voyage, who remarked about tattoos of the high chief Kahekili, which he saw on Maui in November 1778:

> ...is a middle aged man, is rather of a mean appearance, the hair on each side of his head is cut short and a ridge left on the upper part from the forehead to his occiput, this is a common custom among these people, but each side of his head where the hair was off was tattooed in lines forming half circles which I never saw on any other person.

In another interesting and important remark by Samwell in February 1779, he states:

> They are tattawed or marked in various parts; Some have an arm entirely tattawed, others more frequently the Thighs and Legs, the Lines being continued from the upper part of the Thigh to the foot with various figures between them according to their fancy; their bodies are marked with figures of Men and other Animals; Some few among them had one side of their face tattawed, & we saw 2 or 3 who had the whole of the space marked, differing something from the New Zealanders in being done in strait not in spiral Lines. Most of the Chiefs were entirely free from these marks on every part of them, tho' we saw a few who had them, but never any marked on the

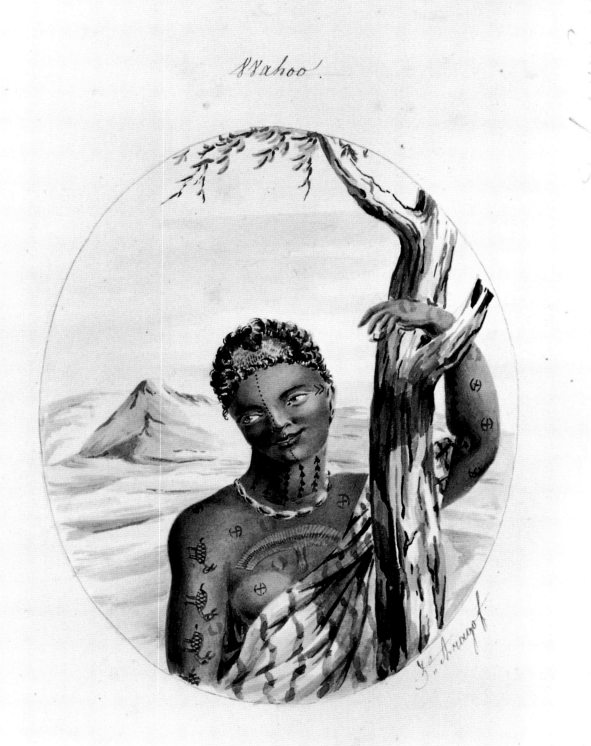

Original ink wash drawing by Jacques Arago entitled "Jeune Fille Des Sandwich" (A Young Woman of the Sandwich Islands). In this picture done in August 1819, a woman is shown with a wide variety of tattoo designs. A fan or *peahi niu* is pictured centered above her breast. Running up the center of her face is a series of dots called *kiko*.* Here the goat tattoos are shown in a style more petroglyph-like. Triangular motifs or *niho mano* run up her neck. *Honolulu Academy of Arts, Gift of Mrs. Frances Damon Holt in memory of John Dominis Holt.*

*This according to the *Hawaiian Dictionary*, Mary Kawena Pukui and Samuel H. Elbert, University of Hawaii Press 1986.

face. This Custom of tattawing seems to be used among these people as a Mortification or at least a rememberance of the dead; Most of those who were tattawed informed us that they bore those Marks in Memory of Ke-owa and Arapai, both great Chiefs & probably the Kings of the island, as the present Heir to the throne of Ouwhaiee, Karipoos' Son, is called after the former; one Man had frequently marks upon him in memory of two or three Chiefs. They seemed to be done in figures agreeable to their own fancy & not so as to distinguish the bearer of them to be a Vassalor dependent on such or such a Chief, for the same device was often found done in memory of different Chiefs, so that it shou'd seem that tho' this custom is almost universal among them it is not imposed upon them as a neccesary duty.

Animal motifs as well as other elements also appear in Hawaiian tattoo art. The artist Arago gives us the most accurate description of this when, in 1819 on his visit, he states that the women:

> ...make drawings of necklaces and garters on the skin in a manner really wonderful: their other devices consist of hunting-horns, helmets, muskets, rings, but more particularly fans and goats, and dominos: together with the name of Tammeamah (Kamehameha), and the day of his death.

Why the goat element appears is still most intriguing. It was Captain Cook who is first credited with bringing goats to the Hawaiian Islands.[10] Because of the novelty and uniqueness of goats to the Hawaiians, they seem to have held them in high regard, hence the abundance of tattoos incorporating their design. It was the Reverend Ellis[11] who describes the goat motif, which seemed to be the favorite design in the 1820s, in much greater detail. It was Makoa, one of Reverend Ellis' guides, who he describes as follows:

> His small eyes were ornamented with tatued vandyke semicircles. Two goats, impressed in the same indelible manner, stood rampant over each of his brows; one, like the supporter of a coat of arms, was fixed on each side of his nose, and two more guarded the corner of his mouth.

With the overthrow of the gods in 1819, tattooing began its gradual decline. The advent of the first missionaries that followed really was the beginning of the end. The practice of tattooing was looked upon by the newly arrived missionaries as pagan and as a reminder of the ancient ways of the Hawaiians' idolatrous past. By the mid-19th century it was no longer practiced and in the 1840s, upon the arrival of the U.S. Exploring Expedition[12] to the islands, the only records of tattoos were of those that contained lettering - usually of the individual wearer. At the end of the 19th century there appear to be only two accounts in literature that relate to old tattoos being seen, both of those on people who were reported to be quite elderly at that time.

Today there is a renaissance of tattooing in the islands. This, along with renewed interest in their native language, culture and arts, is a reflection of the past sure to add to the direction of the future.

Endnotes

[1] This second migration can be traced in traditional chants and recitations (*mele*).
[2] The only indigenous mammal to the Hawaiian group was the bat.
[3] Tamai was probably a fan design, the fan being a symbol of rank of Hawaiian chiefs.
[4] *Kapa* was a type of cloth manufactured through a lengthy process of soaking and beating the bark of the paper mulberry tree. In other parts of Polynesia it is often referred to as *tapa*.
[5] *The Hawaiian Dictionary*, Mary Kawena Pukui and Samuel H. Elbert, University of Hawai`i Press, Honolulu, 1986.
[6] The Hawaiians did not believe in killing the birds that produced the assorted feathers used in making their magnificent feather work. The gum from this nut was used by professional fowlers to ensnare the birds .
[7] Jacques Arago (1790-1855) was the official artist on the scientific French expedition of the ships *L' Uranie* and *L' Physiciennem*, which circumnavigated the world between 1817 and 1820. The commander of the voyage was Louis Claude De Saulses De Freycinet. They recorded many events when they arrived in the islands in 1819.
[8] *Marks of Civilization*, Arnold Rubin editor, Museum of Cultural History, University of California, Los Angeles, 1988.
[9] Upon the death of a person of high rank, great grieving would take place. Some of the more extreme fashions of showing unbounded grief would be self-mutilation, including cutting off fingers, knocking out teeth, cutting hair, etc. In one recorded example in Hawai`i, a woman had her tongue tattooed upon the death of her mother-in-law, Kamamalu, a woman of great rank.
[10] *The Hawaiian Kingdom 1778-1854*, R.S. Kuykendall, The University Press of Hawai`i, Honolulu, 1938.
[11] William Ellis (1794-1872) was a member of the London Missionary Society and spent time in Tahiti as well as Hawai`i and authored several books on Polynesia and Hawai`i. He arrived in Hawai`i in 1822. In 1823 he toured the island of Hawai`i for two months along with Rev. Asa Thurston and Rev. Artemas Bishop and were the first foreigners to ascend the active volcano of Kilauea. His most memorable book *Narrative of a Tour through Hawaii*, published in 1825, notes this observation of goat tattoo motifs.
[12] The U.S. Exploring Expedition under the command of Captain Charles Wilkes (1798-1877) was a scientific expedition to survey the northwest coast of America and the Pacific. The expedition began in 1838 and consisted of five ships. It arrived in the islands in 1841, and teams of scientists explored Oahu, Maui and the island of Hawai`i. Many social and cultural observations are found in the five volumes of the report published in 1845.

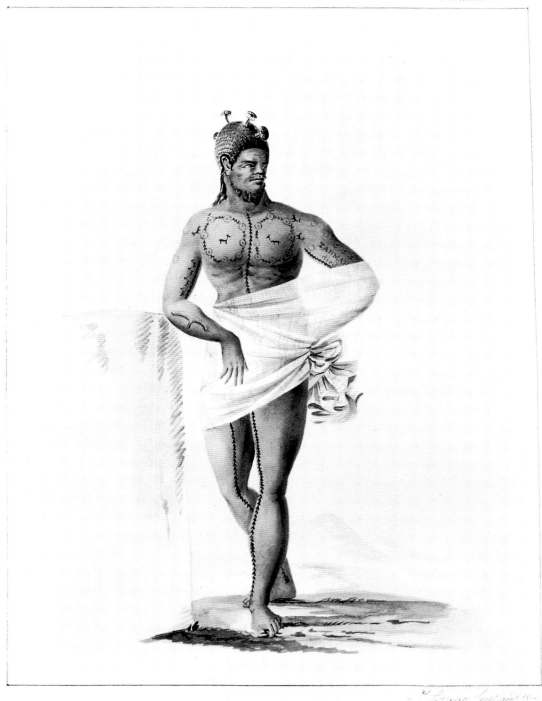

Original ink wash drawing by Jacques Arago entitled "Naturel Des Isles Sandwich" (Native of the Hawaiian Islands). This very famous drawing, done in August 1819, shows a multitude of tattoo motifs including a memorial inscription on his arm relating to the recent death of Kamehameha I. The crescent fan motif or *peahi niu* is seen here on his opposite arm. The breast tattoos are also quite beautiful and unusual and consist of goats surrounded by a circle* and composed of interspersed triangular motifs and circles with what appear to be dots inside. His legs show a classic run of triangular design elements running equally up each side. *Honolulu Academy of Arts, Gift of Mrs. Frances Damon Holt in memory of John Dominis Holt.*
*This circular motif is found in abundance in Hawaiian petroglyph sites.

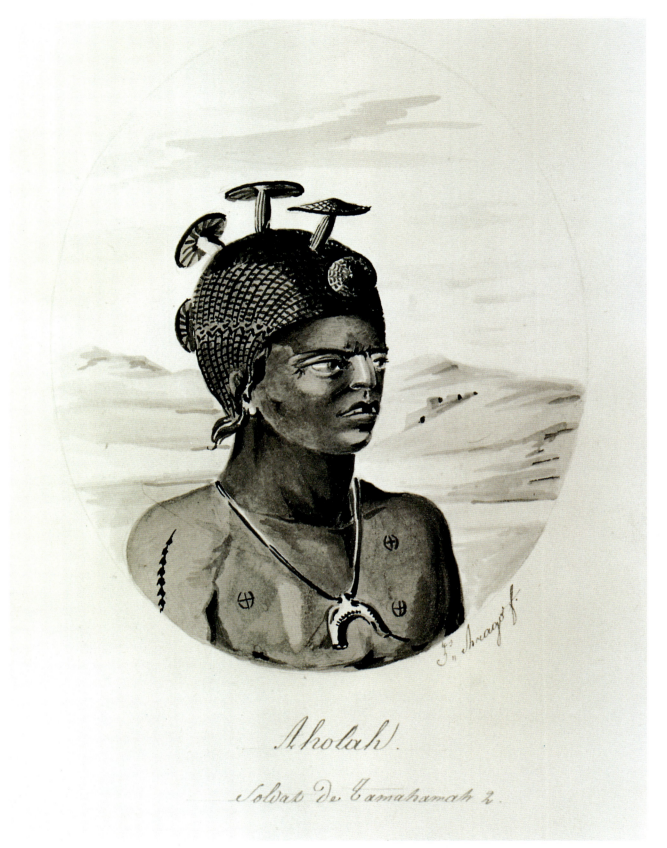

Original ink wash drawing by Jacques Arago entitled "Aholah. Soldat De Tamahahah 2" (Aholah, Warrior of Kamehameha II). In this picture done in August 1819, the warrior Aholah is shown wearing his mushroom-type helmet or *mahiole*. Made of fibers of the *olona* plant, Arago depicted two of these rare types of helmets in the drawings made in Hawai`i while on this expedition. The tattoos shown here are more circular in nature along with triangular motifs running up the shoulder. Some people regard this triangular design as being inspired by shark teeth. This shark tooth design, when found on tapa beaters and stamps, is known as *niho mano*. Honolulu Academy of Arts, Gift of Mrs. Frances Damon Holt in memory of John Dominis Holt.

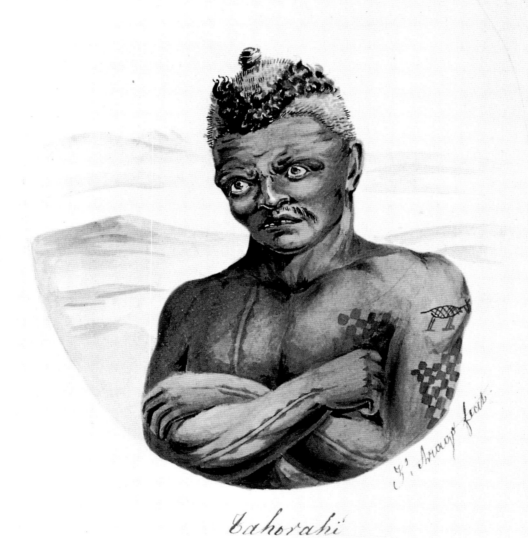

Original ink wash drawing by Jacques Arago entitled "Tahorahi." In this picture done in August 1819, the classic "checkerboard" pattern is shown on the breast and arm. This motif, known as *papa konane* in Hawaiian, was one of the principal design elements recorded by the early explorers in the 18th century at the time of contact. One of the more unusual renderings of what appears to be a goat or horse is seen here in a style more in the manner of a petroglyph than a tattoo.
Honolulu Academy of Arts, Gift of Mrs. Frances Damon Holt in memory of John Dominis Holt.

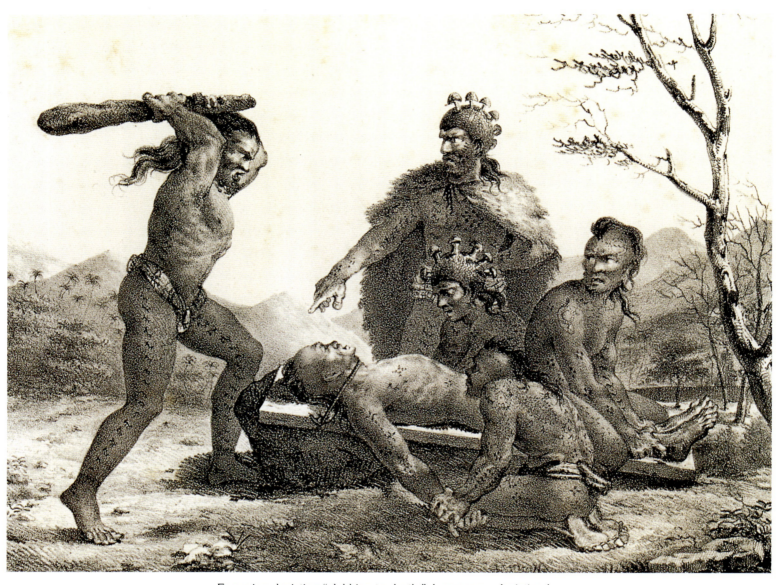
Engraving depicting "clubbing to death." A gruesome depiction by the artist Jacques Arago, who sketched this scene in Hawai`i in 1819. It has been included here to show the abundance of tattoo motifs present on Hawaiians at the time.

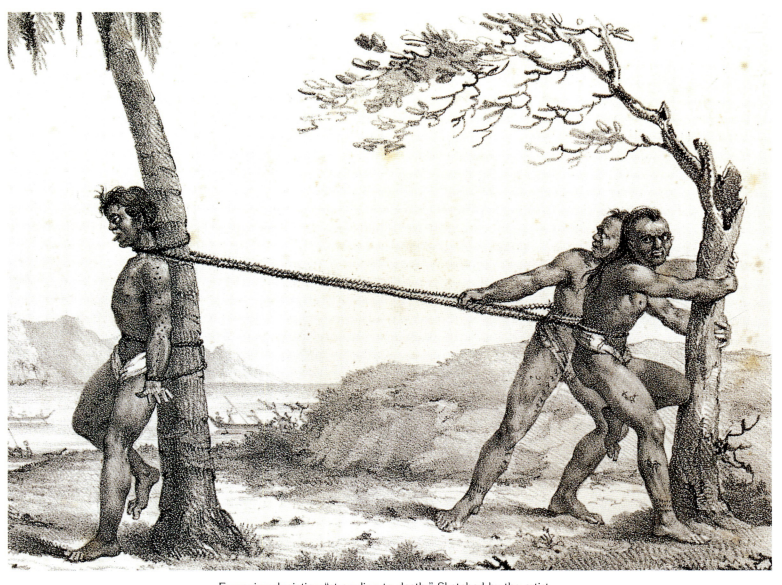

Engraving depicting "strangling to death." Sketched by the artist Jacques Arago, it is included here to show the abundance of tattoo motifs seen at the time. One year later, in 1820, Hawaiian society would be changed forever with the arrival of the first missionaries from Boston.

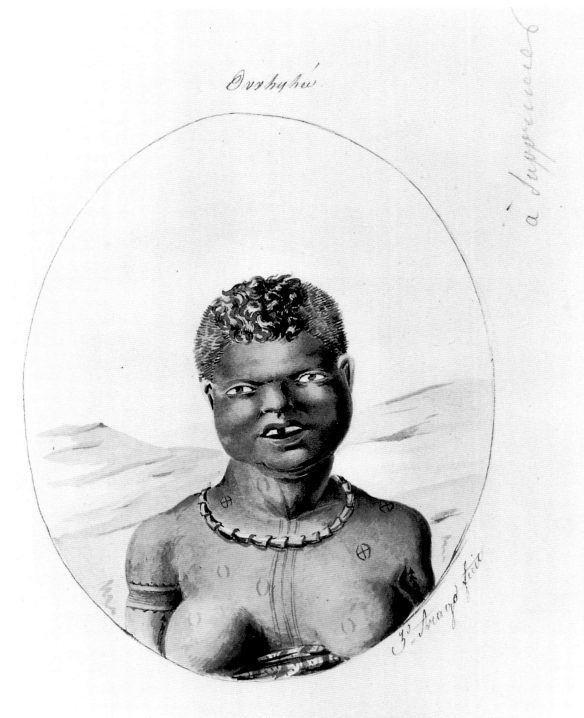

Original ink wash drawing by Jacques Arago entitled "Une Des Veves De Tamahmah 1er" (One of the Widows of Kamehameha I). In this picture done in August 1819, the widow is shown missing her two front teeth, undoubtedly knocked out by her as a sign of grief at her husband's recent death. The tattoos accurately record Arago's written description at the time, consisting of armbands, lines between the breasts and circles with what appear to be crosses. *Honolulu Academy of Arts, Gift of Mrs. Frances Damon Holt in memory of John Dominis Holt.*

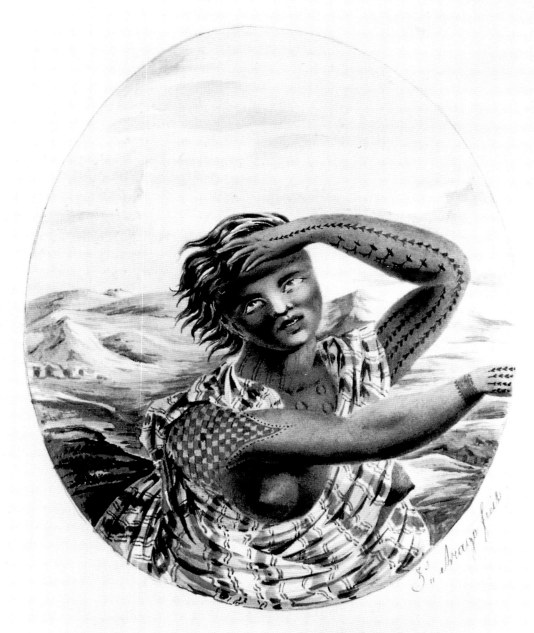

Original ink wash drawing by Jacques Arago entitled "Taimoorah… Jeune Fille Dansant" (Young Girl Dancing). In this picture done in August 1819, Arago has captured what he termed his "domino motif" apparent on the girl's shoulder as well as other typical design elements including a repetitive design of goats on her forearm. *Honolulu Academy of Arts, Gift of Mrs. Frances Damon Holt in memory of John Dominis Holt.*

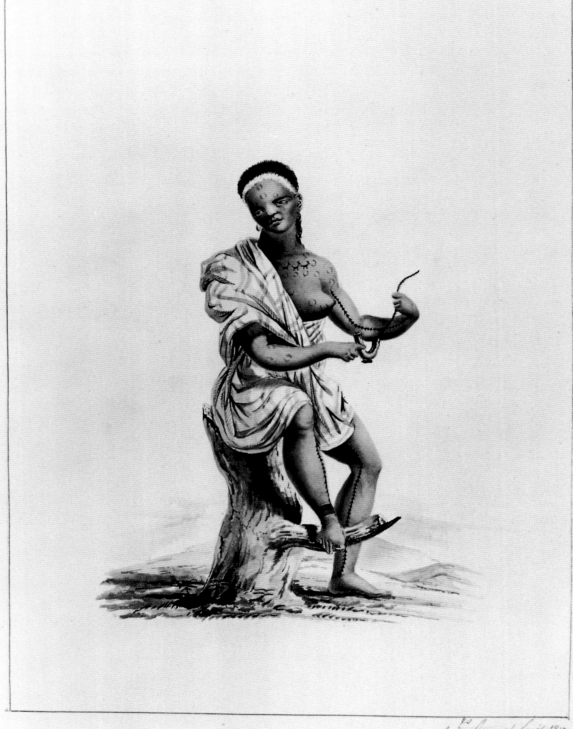

Original ink wash drawing by Jacques Arago entitled "Irini, Femmes Des Isles Sandwich" (Irini, Woman of the Sandwich Islands). In this picture done in August 1819, Irini is shown holding a pipe in her hand. Her tattoos consist of goats above breasts, circles on face and breasts and triangular motifs running up the legs and arms. *Honolulu Academy of Arts, Gift of Mrs. Frances Damon Holt in memory of John Dominis Holt.*

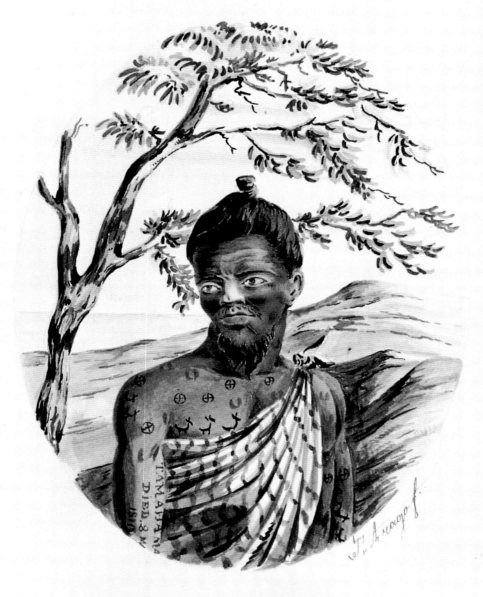

Original ink wash drawing by Jacques Arago entitled "Lahihenahou, Une Des Officiers Du Roi" (Lahihenahou, One of the Officers of the King). In this picture done in August 1819, Lahihenahou is shown wearing a wide variety of tattoo motifs including memorial, goats, circles, etc. *Honolulu Academy of Arts, Gift of Mrs. Frances Damon Holt in memory of John Dominis Holt.*

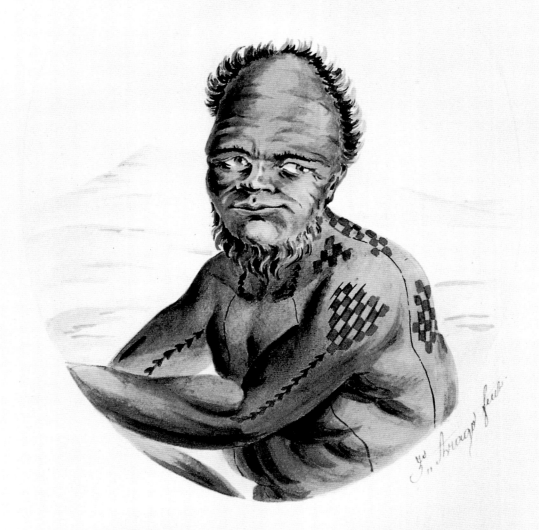

102

Original ink wash drawing by Jacques Arago entitled "Aho. Naturel De Mowhee" (Aho, native of Maui). This picture, done in August 1819, shows the checkerboard pattern *papa konane* along with the triangular motif running up the arms. *Honolulu Academy of Arts, Gift of Mrs. Frances Damon Holt in memory of John Dominis Holt.*

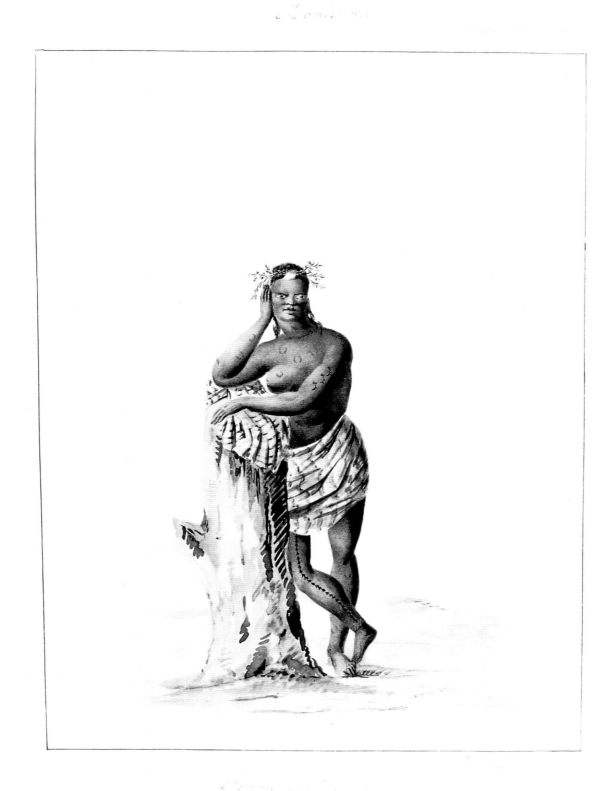

Original ink wash drawing by Jacques Arago entitled "Femme Des Iles Sandwich" (Woman of the Sandwich Islands). In this picture done in August 1819, the artist Arago has accurately drawn a woman of the time period. Dressed in a *kapa* or barkcloth wrap, she is depicted wearing a wide variety of tattoo motifs of the time period. *Honolulu Academy of Arts, Gift of Mrs. Frances Damon Holt in memory of John Dominis Holt.*

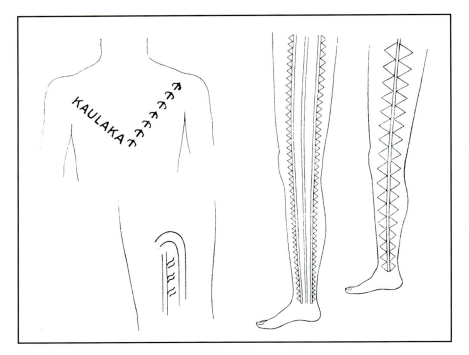

Drawing of Hawaiian tattoo motifs. This is one of the last known depictions of tattoo on living persons and was recorded by Professor Augustin Kramer in 1897 on the island of Hawai`i. From his book entitled *Hawai`i, Ostmikronesien und Samoa*, published in Stuttgart in 1906.

Engraving depicting a Hawaiian woman. This is a depiction after the artist Jacques Arago, who sketched the original drawing in 1819. A rather fanciful portrayal of traditional Hawaiian tattooing with a lot of artistic license. Published in the 1840s from a "popular" French edition of Pacific Voyages.

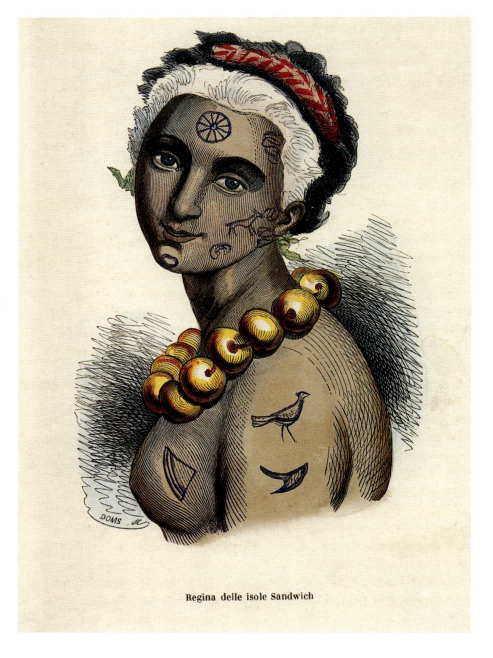

Regina delle isole Sandwich

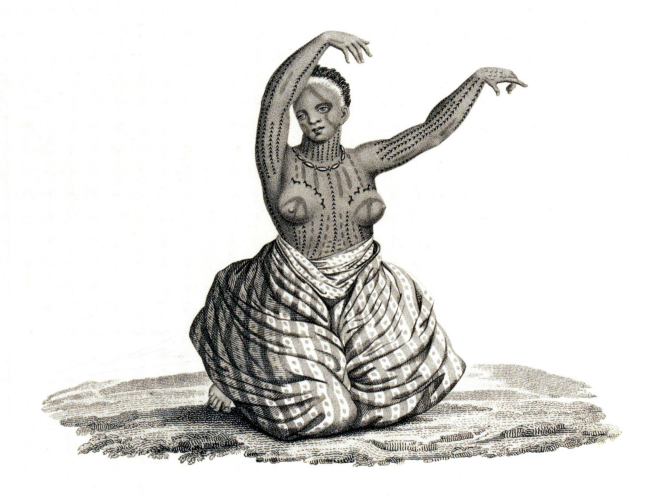

ÎLES SANDWICH: FEMME DE L'ÎLE MOWI DANSANT.

Engraving entitled "Isles Sandwich: Femme De L'ile Mowi Dansant." In this wonderful picture sketched in 1819, the artist Jacques Arago records an unusual design motif with a representation of goats tattooed around the breasts. Often referred to as the "Venus" of Hawai`i, it is a striking and poignant depiction of a Hula Dancer who appears dressed in a *kapa* skirt.

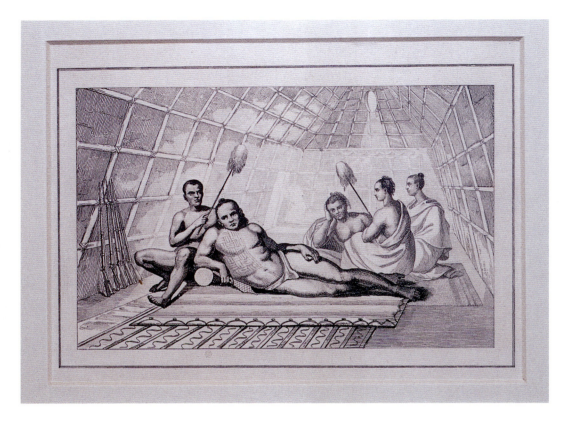

Engraving depicting a chief reclining. This is an image after the artist Louis Choris, who sketched the original drawing in Hawai`i in 1816. This print shows a good representation of chest tattoo as observed by Choris.

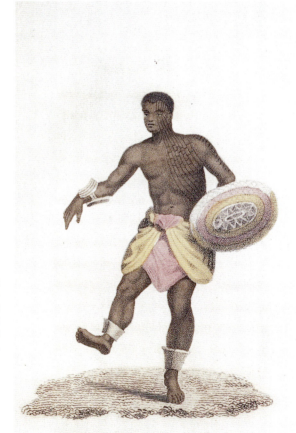

Engraving entitled "Dancer of the Sandwich Islands." From *The World in Miniature – South Sea Islands*, published in 1824 in London, Frederick Shorbel editor. A depiction after the artist Louis Choris, who sketched the original drawing in 1816.

106

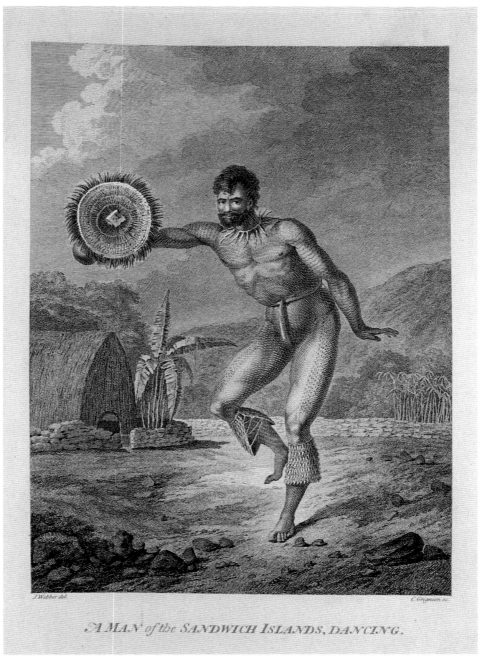

Engraving entitled "A Man of the Sandwich Islands, Dancing." Published in the atlas to Cook's third and final fateful voyage, this drawing is by John Webber and is the first known depiction of tattoo on a Hawaiian.

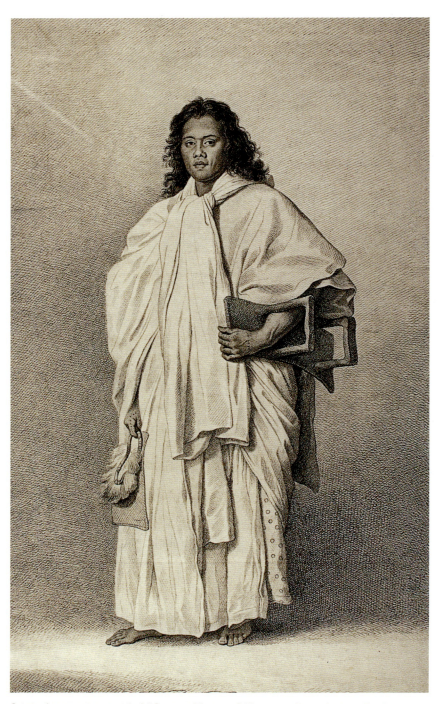

Original engraving entitled "Omai a Native of Ulaietea...Brought into England in 1774 by Tobias Furneauz Esq. Commander of his Majesty's Sloop Adventure humbly inscribed to the Right Hon.ble John Earl of Sandwich, First Commisioner for executing the Office of Lord High Admiral of Great Britain and Ireland etc. etc. By his Lordship most devoted Servant Fra. Bartolozzi, published according to Act of Parl. 25th Oct 1774."

Omai was from the island of Ra'iatea and, with some misgivings from Captain Cook, boarded the ship *Adventure* under the command of Lieutenant Furneaux, serving as an interpreter for the remainder of Cook's second voyage. At the end of 1773 Cook's own ship, the *Resolution*, became separated from Furneaux's by a violent storm; whereas Cook continued his voyage, the *Adventure* headed home for England. So it was in 1774 the first "Noble Savage" arrived in London, almost by accident. He soon became the toast of London society, having an audience with the King and attending balls and hunts. He spent two years in England, returning back to Tahiti on Cook's third voyage to a hero's welcome and a multitude of gifts. In this engraving he is shown dressed wearing a barkcloth toga with tattoos on his hands. Omai was the first tattooed Polynesian to set foot on English soil.

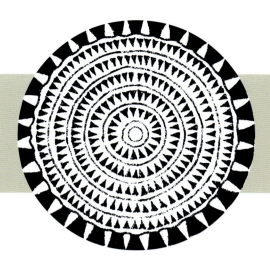

TAHITI

The word Tahiti is used to cover a geographic triangle formed by the Society-Cook-Austral complex of islands, the cultures all being closely related. This area consists of the Austral Islands to the south, the Cook Islands to the west, the Gambier Islands to the east and the islands of Tahiti lying at the top. The islands of Tahiti will be the main focus of this chapter. Naturally forming two areas, the windward islands of this group are formed by the principal island of Tahiti, along with Mo'orea, Me'etia, Tetiaroa (Marlon Brando's private island) and Mai'ao, with the leeward islands being comprised of Ra'iatea, Taha'a, Huaheine, Bora Bora, Tubuai and Maupiti. All the islands, with the exceptions of Tetiaroa and Tubuai, are "high islands" with a volcanic core surrounded by barrier coral reefs. Continual erosion has produced a well-watered terrain on the majority of the islands, with Mount Orohena on Tahiti the highest and most dramatic peak, measuring in height over 7,000 feet.

The climate is warm and humid with an average temperature of 85 degrees Fahrenheit. Rainfall varies according to altitude and coastal position with the windward islands receiving well over 100 inches per year, creating a lush environment. Due to the richness of the earth a wide variety of plants were cultivated, including taro and sweet potatoes with breadfruits or *uru* being the main staple.[1] Meat was eaten only on ceremonial occasions by those of high rank and was limited to pork and the occasional dog or fowl.

The islands of Tahiti were settled from the Marquesas, with a settlement date of approximately 600 AD. Evidence of development within this area, along with a later dispersal to other local Polynesian groups, is shown by the archaeological remains of the tanged reversed triangular adze blade along with a similarity in other objects showing regional variations - all being based upon a common theme.

Tahitian society at the time of contact consisted of three main, distinct classes: The high chiefs or *ari'i* at the top; the middle class or *ra'atira* composed of farmers, landed gentry, warriors, and administrators; and the *manahune* - the oppressed commoners.[2] An unusual group known as the *arioi* society existed in a periphery of these classes; its members, travelling players, were devoted to entertaining the entire population.[3] This group, which was unique to the Society Islands, enjoyed a tremendous amount of notoriety when the first Europeans reported their activities. The missionaries despised their canoe-wandering habits, along with their sexual license and eroticism. The fact that they were obliged to destroy their offspring or resign their membership did not help matters, either. Known for their locust-like rapacity that often desolated entire districts, many Tahitians were forced to move inland to be out of reach of the *arioi*.

Religious beliefs centered around ritual worship of a pantheon of gods and ancestral spirits, with the cult of *Oro* closely linked to the *arioi* society, the other deities being *Tane, Ro'o, Tu* and *Ta'aroa*. Due to a shift in political powers beginning around the time of contact, *Oro*, the son of *Ta'aroa*, became the most important god with the help of priests at Opoa in Ra'iatea. Taking the place of the god *Ta'aroa*, the change was a bloody one, with the *Oro* faction removing all opposition. The symbol of the god *Oro*, the god of war, was installed at the temple or *marae* at Taputapuatea on the island of Ra'iatea in the late 18th century.[4] This cult reigned supreme until Pomare I decided to adopt Christianity around 1820. Like other areas of Polynesia, *tapu* regulations were always present with a set of strict guidelines governing both secular and non-secular activities.

Settlements consisted of small groups of houses or hamlets set in shady areas along the coast. Here Tahitians lived in houses or *fare*, their households consisting of one room, rectangular in shape with square or oval ends. The roofs were thatched of coconut fronds or pandanus, the sides composed of upright bamboo, with a nearby cooking hut or *fare tutu* used by the women for earth-oven cooking.

Domestic crafts were varied, with barkcloth or *tapa* manufacture being an integral part of the fiber arts that involved women of all grades. Specialist craftsmen or *tahu'a* followed other artistic pursuits such as carving fine wooden seats, flywhisks, spears and other possessions that symbolized high rank. Canoes were also an important part of Tahitian society, being made by these specialist craftsmen. Canoes consisting of two types were constructed, with the *pahi* the most important and elaborate. These were impressive, deep-keeled ships made of many planks with stages set above the hulls for fighting.[5]

Clothing in Tahitian society consisted of a simple loin cloth or *maro* for males, with a wrap-around *pareu* or waist cloth worn by both sexes - all being fashioned from

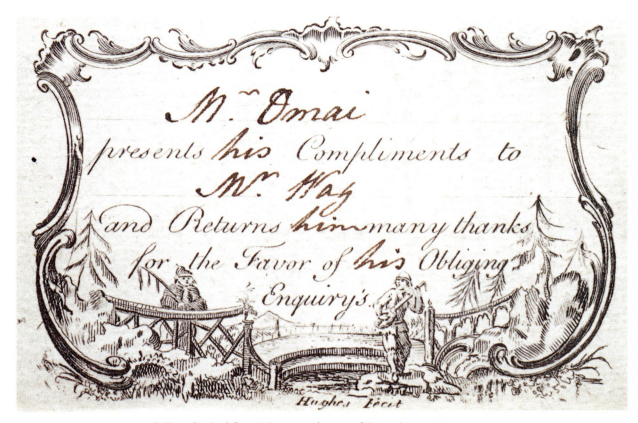

Calling Card of Omai. A rare and unusual item given out to London society and other notable people he encountered.

barkcloth. Decorated barkcloth ponchos, as well as fine mats, also were occasionally worn.[6] Large toga-like cloaks were produced – with the quality of all clothing and tattooing indicating his or her social status. Persons of high rank wore ritual loincloths on special occasions, these being decorated with the precious red or yellow feathers of birds.

The first European to set foot on the island of Tahiti was the Englishman Samuel Wallis (1728-1795) with his ship *Dolphin* anchoring on June 17, 1767, at Taiarapu on the southern end of the island. It was not a pleasant encounter, as the natives became so hostile that he was forced to intimidate them by firing his cannons. The next day Wallis moved his ship to Matavai Bay and was immediately surrounded by thousands of Tahitians in their canoes. Almost at once the ship was besieged under a hail of spears and stones forcing Wallis to fire his cannons once again. The next day he sent an armed crew to shore to take official possession of the island, but was attacked immediately again. Deciding once and for all to put an end to this behavior, he fired his cannons at the canoes and the crowd gathered on shore, resulting in numerous victims.[7] While the wounded were being lamented over, Wallis sent a crew ashore to destroy all the canoes in the area. Now being much more submissive, the islanders began cooperating and helping the English refurbish the ship all in exchange for nails.

The next European visitor to Tahiti was the French Captain Louis Antoine de Bougainville (1729- 1811), whose two ships *Etoile* and *Boudeuse* sighted the island on April 2, 1768, only a few months after the visit of Wallis. It was Bougainville, who so loved and was loved by the Tahitian people, who gave credence to the myth of the "Noble Savage."[8] To quote from his journal,

> I feel as though I have been transported to the Garden of Eden. Everywhere finding hospitality, peace, inner joy with every appearance of happiness. What a country! What a people!

This visit was not as peaceful and pleasant as it appeared, with a Tahitian being shot dead and three natives bayoneted, infuriating Bougainville.[9]

When Wallis returned to England, the Admiralty had already decided to send a new expedition to the Pacific to observe the transit of Venus[10] across the sun on June 3, 1769, with the result being the first of Captain Cook's voyages. While on this voyage, he visited Tahiti, discovering the leeward group, naming them the Society Islands in honor of the Royal Society in London. Cook visited the islands on subsequent voyages, doing away with many of the myths and illusions of his predecessors. The results were impressive, leaving us with valuable collections and records, both literary and graphic, making it the most important source today on ancient Tahiti.[11]

Foreign vessels continued using Matavai Bay and Tahiti for a favorable anchorage, with the local chief Tu becoming increasingly more powerful and embarking on wars with his neighbors. With the assistance of Captain Bligh (1754-1817) in 1788 and of his mutineers in 1790, Tu was able to subdue his rivals. Tu, under the new name Pomare, assumed control of the whole island and established himself in hereditary chieftainship, being succeeded by his son in 1803. A series of wars firmly established the dynasty in 1815 and formed alliances with the leeward islands. The Pomare dynasty continued until 1877 ending with Pomare IV. The French assumed control of the group in 1842, under Queen Pomare's reign, with the formal annexing of the windward islands in 1880.[12]

Without a doubt the most profound influence on the native culture was that of the missionaries, with the advent of the London Missionary Society (Protestant) arriving in 1797. Over the next several decades mission stations were set up on the majority of the islands.[13] Within a short period of time the combined zeal of both the converter and converted swept away any remnants of traditional religious and ceremonial life, with the exception of the language, which is still alive today, being heard on the crowded and congested streets of Papeete. Today the Tahitian people face numerous challenges with an extremely high cost of living and a burgeoning population resulting in extreme poverty in some areas. The principal sources of income for the islands are black pearls, copra, vanilla and tourism. Tourism has also suffered in recent years, this due in part to a boycott launched in protest of French nuclear testing on nearby Muraroa atoll. Artist Paul Gauguin, one of Tahiti's most famous residents, may have summed up the situation best when, in 1896, he made the following statement about the continued desecration made by the white man:

> There used to be many strange and beautiful things here, but no trace of them now remains. The natives have nothing to do, and think of one thing only, drinking. There is much prostitution. Day by day the race vanishes...they are dying of despair.

Tahitian Tattoo – *tatau*

The art of tattooing in Tahiti was a tradition that originated among the gods who considered it to be ornamental and pleasing, according to the Reverend William Ellis. Based upon a legend in Tahitian mythology, a child was born after a union between Apouvaru and Ta'aroa resulting in the birth of a child known as Matamata-arahu (Printer in Charcoal). Being seduced by her brothers, they invented *tatau* in order to attract her. Being jealously guarded by her mother, she slipped away in order to be tattooed only to fall victim to the sexual desires of her brothers. Thus the supernatural origin of Tahitian tattooing, with Matamat-arahu and Tu Ra'i Po becoming the patron spirits of the art. At the beginning of the tattooing process the professional tattoo artists known as *tatatau* or *tahu'a tatau* would offer prayers to these two spirits to ensure the operation's success and that the patterns would attract numerous admirers. Carved images of these two gods were kept by the tattoo artist in the *marae* of their district and consulted prior to the operation.

Men and women of all ranks were tattooed in a series of operations that began at puberty, occasionally continuing on in stages for many years to come. It was Sir Joseph Banks, the naturalist on Cook's first voyage, who leaves us with one of the more detailed descriptions of design and motif elements:

> ...everyone is markd thus in different parts of his body according may to his humour or different circumstances in life. Some have ill designd figures of men, birds, or dogs, but they more generally have this figure Z either simply, as the women are generally markd with it, on every Joint of their fingers and toes and often round the outside of their feet, or in different figures of it as square, circles, crescents, &c. which both sexes have on their arms and leggs; in short they have an infinite diversity of figures in which they place this mark and some of them we were told had significations but this we never learnt to our satisfaction. Their faces are in general left without any marks, I did not see more than one instance to the contrary." He later goes on to say: "Tho they are so various in the application of the fingers I have mentiond that both the quanity and situation of them seems to depend intirely upon the humour of each individual, yet all the Islanders I have seen (except those of Ohiteroa{Rurutu}) agree in having all their buttocks covered with a deep black; over this most have arches drawn one over another as high as their short ribbs, which are often ¼ of an inch broad and neatly worked on their edges with indenttions &c. These arches are their great pride, both men and women shew them with great pleasure whether as a beauty or proof of their perseverance and resolution in bearing pain I can not tell, as the pain of doing this is almost intolerable especially the arches upon the loins which are so much more susceptible to pain than the fleshy buttocks.

Men, it appears, were more extensively tattooed than women, with certain patterns reserved for those of high rank. The most important tattoo, the blackening of the buttocks,[14] was the first one acquired at the onset of puberty. At the time of contact some tattoos had ritual or ceremonial significance with special markings reserved for the *arioi* society and members of high rank.

Due to decades of European contact, new design elements started appearing, described by the missionary William Ellis in the 1820s:

> From the lower part of the back, a number of straight, waved or zigzag lines, rise in the direction of the spine and branch off regularly towards the shoulders. But, of the upper part of the body, the chest is the most tataued. Every variety of figure is seen here: coca-nut and bread-fruit trees, with convolvolus wreaths hanging round them, boys gathering fruit, men engaged in battle, in the manual exercises, triumphing by a fallen foe; or as I have frequently seen it, they are represented as carrying a human sacrifice to the temple. Every kind of animal—goats, dogs, fowls, and fish—may at times be seen on this part of the body; muskets, swords, pistols, clubs, spears, and other weapons of war, are also stamped upon their arms or chest.

As in other areas of Polynesia, tattooing was prohibited by the missionaries on all their converts but was so deeply engrained in Tahitian society that the missionaries resorted to severe measures to prevent illicitly acquired tattoos from appearing.[15]

Like most other areas in Polynesia, the actual technique used in smooth-skin tattooing was similar, the most accurate account left to us by Frederick Bennett who, in 1834, had his upper arm tattooed:[16]

> While at this island (Ra'iatea), I gratified a wish to observe and effects of the tattoo by having a figure thus impressed upon myself. The artist I engaged was a Tahitian; and from the numerous patterns displayed on his person we selected a circular figure, named pote; the spot I preferred devoting to the impression was the upper arm. The operation commenced by bending the elastic rib of a cocoa-nut leaf into a circular form, and smearing its edge with a black fluid composed of the lamp black of burned candle-nuts diluted to the consistence of printer's ink. This placed on the skin marked the outer circle; to execute which by the eye along would have proved difficult task; the remainder of the design, however was completed without any similar guide. The tatooing instrument, a thin plate of boars tusk, about half an inch in breadth, sharply toothed at its margin, and fixed, at an angle to the extremity of a slender handle, was then imbued with the black fluid, and made to penetrate the skin by striking short and quick strokes on its handle with a second and heavier piece of wood, of conical form; the artist desisting after every few taps, to wipe away the ink and oozing blood, that he might observe better the effect produced and the line to follow. In less than one hour the design was completed. The pain produced by the operation was rather annoying than severe. It was only felt during the application of the toothed instument, when the sensation was of a dull pricking nature, hard to endure when long protracted and felt much more sensitively in some parts of the skin than in others. The bleeding from the punctures was trifling at first; but as the work proceeded, and the stimulus determined the blood more freely to the surface, each application of the instrument was attended with a greater flow. The arm continued inflamed, and a red serum oozed from the puncture for several hours; but on the following day the part was merely tender, and the redness of the skin had given place to a bruised appearnce, extending to the elbow; (an effect of course not perceptible in the dark skin of the native) while the effused serum gave the tattooed figure a varnished appearnce. In four days the arm was perfectly well; and the scarf skin peeling off, left the tattooed marks beneath of a bright blue colour and slightly elevated...The operation of tattooing is not always followed by these mild results: in some robust Europeans, whose curiosity has induced them to submit to the process, I have witnessed very severe

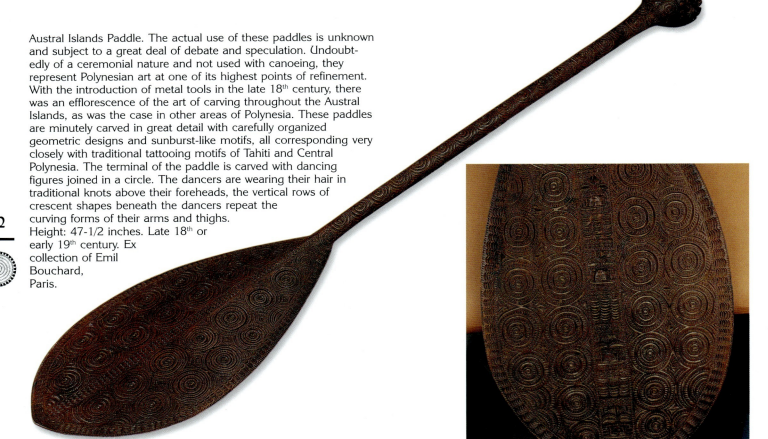

Austral Islands Paddle. The actual use of these paddles is unknown and subject to a great deal of debate and speculation. Undoubtedly of a ceremonial nature and not used with canoeing, they represent Polynesian art at one of its highest points of refinement. With the introduction of metal tools in the late 18th century, there was an efflorescence of the art of carving throughout the Austral Islands, as was the case in other areas of Polynesia. These paddles are minutely carved in great detail with carefully organized geometric designs and sunburst-like motifs, all corresponding very closely with traditional tattooing motifs of Tahiti and Central Polynesia. The terminal of the paddle is carved with dancing figures joined in a circle. The dancers are wearing their hair in traditional knots above their foreheads, the vertical rows of crescent shapes beneath the dancers repeat the curving forms of their arms and thighs.
Height: 47-1/2 inches. Late 18th or early 19th century. Ex collection of Emil Bouchard, Paris.

effects insue; the inflamed skin passing into a state of suppuration; though it is curious to know how far the latter effect, and even ulceration will extend, without the integrity of the tattooed figure being materially impaired.

Though the previous account was performed several decades after the appearance of Christianity, with the art in full decline, it still provides us with a very detailed account of the actual procedure, the only difference being the elaborate amount of ritual that would have followed every step of the operation prior to contact with the Europeans.

Today the art of tattooing is making a comeback in Tahiti with a wide repertoire of designs drawn from both Marquesan as well as traditional Tahitian motifs. This seems a very a fitting new beginning to a once flourishing art form and a tribute to the word *tatau* itself… a word shared with the rest of the world as tattoo.

Eight Hierarchial Orders of The Arioi Society as Recorded by Henry with Identifying Tattoo Markings

FIRST ORDER, being the highest who resided over all of the rest: a man for the men and a woman for the women, they were called *arioi maro 'ura* or comedians of the red loin girdle. Or they were called *avae parai,* translated as besmeared legs, because most of them were tattooed completely black from their feet up to their groins, though some limited the operation to the knee.
SECOND ORDER, termed *harotea* or light print, had filigree bars cross-wise on both sides of the body from the armpits downwards towards the front.
THIRD ORDER, termed *taputu* or *haaputu,* translated as pile-to-gether, had diversified curves and lines radiating upwards towards the sides from the lower end of the dorsal column to the middle of the back.
FOURTH ORDER, termed *otiore* or unfinished, had light prints upon their knuckles and wrists with heavier ones upon their arms and shoulders.
FIFTH ORDER, termed *hua* or small, had two or three small points upon each shoulder.
SIXTH ORDER, termed *atoro* or stripe, had one small stripe down the left side.
SEVENTH ORDER, termed *ohemara* or seasoned-bamboo, had a circle around the ankle.
EIGHTH ORDER, termed *tara-tutu* or pointed thorn, had small marks in the hollows of the knees.

Endnotes

[1] Breadfruit or *uru* was the main staple of the Tahitian diet and was prepared either baked in earth ovens or pounded into paste, occasionally mixed with coconut milk. It was the mission of the ill-fated Captain William Bligh whose job it was to bring this "perfect food" back to the West Indies as a source of cheap, easily cultivated sustenance for the then-burgeoning slave population. While returning from Tahiti on this official voyage, the mutiny of the *Bounty* took place on April 28, 1789, near the island of Tofua in the Ha'apai group Tonga.
[2] Another intermediary class known as the *laotai* existed between the *ari'i* and *ra'atira,* occasionally creating a kind of nobility by intermarriage. Slaves were known as *ofeofe.*
[3] Their chants and dances served to perpetuate traditions, passing these traditions from one generation to the next.
[4] This temple, sometimes known as the "International Temple" of the islands of Tahiti, was a rectangular area covered with paving stones and surrounded by low walls. At one end stood the altar or *ahu* in the form of a graded pyramid. Stones were placed upright in front of the altar within the walled areas symbolizing the genealogies of the creators of the *marae*. Human sacrifices took place on these many *maraes* of Tahiti.
[5] These large "war canoes" were propelled by paddlers who did not partake in the initial fighting.
[6] Barkcloth or *tapa* in Tahiti was decorated with patterns painted in freehand in various colors or with the impressions of fern leaves dipped in brown pigment and then pressed onto the cloth.
[7] Wallis named the island of Tahiti "King George III Island."
[8] Once back in France, Bougainville promoted Tahiti's idyllic image, giving her the name "La Nouvelle Cythere," and at the same time proclaiming the islands to be a French possession. His published account entitled *Voyage*, released in 1771, was a resounding and long-lasting success. It was this book that the French philosophers Jean-Jacques Rousseau (1712-1778) and Denis Diderot (1713-1784) drew upon to create the myth of the "Noble Savage," with Diderot stating: "This is the first time my reading has tempted me to visit a country other than my own."
[9] In an argument over the price of a pig, three natives were bayoneted to death with Bougainville immediately demanding that justice be done. The four soldiers were arrested, covering up for each other, making it impossible to prove which one of them had done the actual murders. Bougainville then ordered the drawing of lots to decide which one of them would be hanged. However, salvation came at the last moment when the Tahitians, hearing of this punishment, pleaded with the Captain to release them, the natives saying: "Though you kill us, we are still your friends."
[10] The observations were a failure due to the lack of precision in his instruments.
[11] Captain Cook was the first mariner to map the whole Pacific Ocean as a result of his three voyages of discovery. His maps of some island groups are still in use today.
[12] The leeward group was under the nominal control of native governments until 1888.
[13] The Tahitian people suffered terribly from the internal wars and introduced diseases of the 18th century, the population falling from around 125,000 people at the time of Cook to about 8,000 in 1815.
[14] Sir Joseph Banks observed that it was performed on both sexes between the ages of 14 and 18. He also stated that he never saw one single person of a mature age without a buttock tattoo. It was the elder Forster, of Cook's voyage, who recorded the following names for design elements of buttock tattoo: The solid blackened in area was named *taomaro*, the arches, *avari*.
[15] In a rather strange twist to this situation, the artist Paul Gauguin recorded the tattooing of Tahitians by missionaries to mark them as social outcasts for deeds done against the church: "Near her stood a woman a hundred years old, an ancestor of hers. Her ghastly decrepitude was the more terrible for her show of perfect cannibal teeth…On her cheek was a tattoo, a dark mark of uncertain shape, like a letter of the Latin alphabet…I had already seen many tattoos, but none like this; this one was certainly European. I was told that the missionaries, in their campaign against lubricity, had imprinted certain women with a sign of infamy, and admonition of hell. This filled them with shame - not because of the sin they had committed, but because of the ridicule and approbrium attracted by that sign of destruction."
[16] Frederick Bennett's accounts were published in 1840 in his book entitled *Narrative of a Whaling Voyage Round the Globe, from the year 1833-36.*

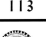

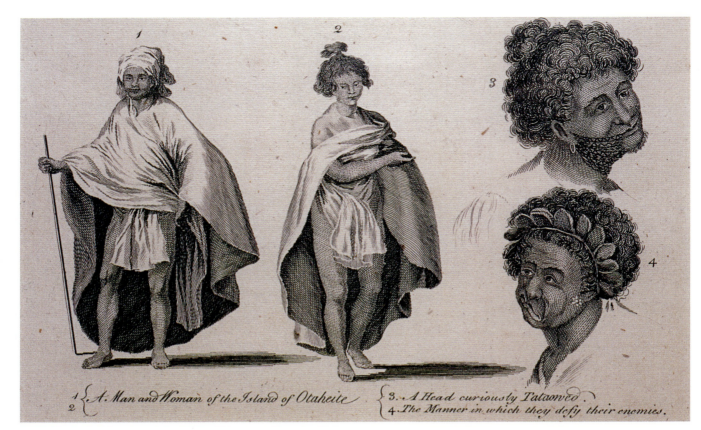

Engraving entitled "A Man and Woman of the Island of Otaheite." From Parkinson's journal published in 1784. Sydney Parkinson was employed by Sir Joseph Banks and accompanied him on Captain Cook's first voyage as a botanical draftsman. In this unusual print, labeled as item #3 is an illustration of Tahitian facial tattooing, one of the few 18th century depictions known to exist. How accurate a portrayal it is remains unknown.

Engraving entitled "Te po a Chief of Raratonga." Frontispiece to *A Narrative of Missionary Enterprises in the South Sea Islands* by Reverend John Williams. Raratonga is the principal island of the Cook group and lies south-southwest of the island of Tahiti. This illustration published in 1837 depicts the principal chief of the island complete with all his regalia and tattoos.

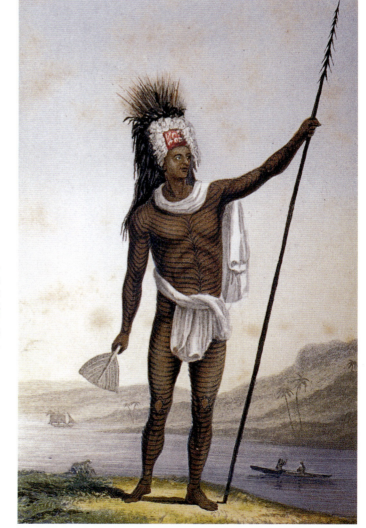

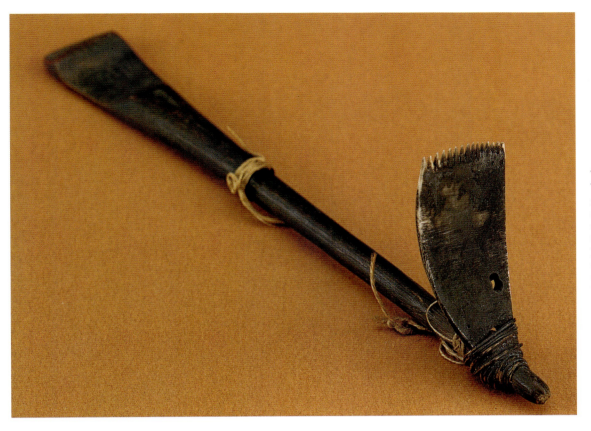

Tattooing needle or comb. Termed *uhi*, these are masterpieces of design and construction. Possibly collected on one of Captain Cook's voyages. Length: 4-5/8 inches. Ex collection of Warwick Castle, John Hewett, and Lord McAlpine of London.

Original watercolor of tattoo patterns and tools. The woman depicted in this picture is shown with a variety of traditional Tahitian tattoo motifs, although the accumulation of patterns shown here on the body is most unlikely. In the lower right is a depiction of a man from the Tuamotu Islands, the checkerboard patterns being used in this area of low lying atolls to mark and distinguish valiant warriors. The upper right corner depicts a man from the island of Mangareva with the specific patterns shown here being recorded by the voyage of Captain Dumont d' Urville. The tools depicted at the top are a tattooing comb and small mallet. Watercolor by Jean-Louis Saquet.

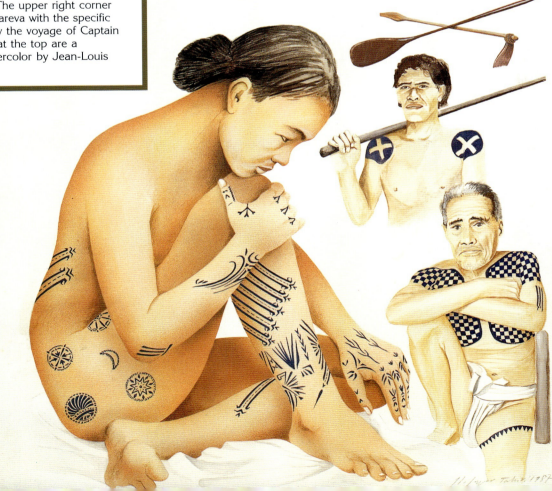

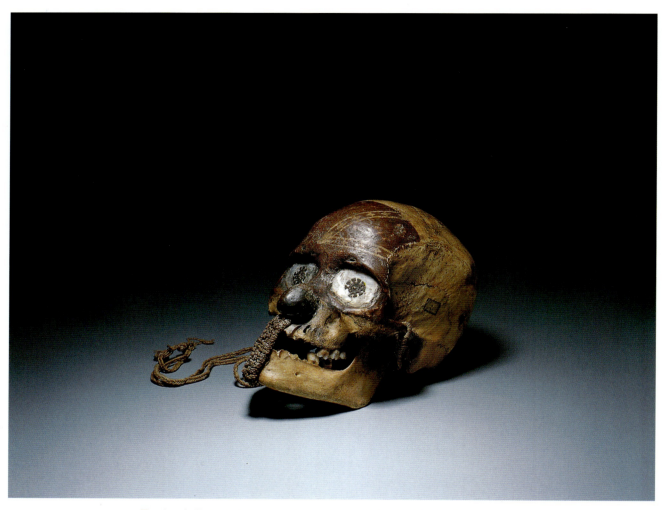

Trophy skull. A skull from the head of a powerful enemy, these were often carried into battle attached to a woven fiber belt at the waist. Skulls represent the most sacred part of the body and were imbued with much *mana,* thus protecting the warrior in battle. In this example, a tattoo design element known as *hiku-pona* is present and is painted on the forehead of the skull. The paint appears to be red ochre and is sacred in nature. The eyes are pearl shell with cut out turtle shell plaques. The nose is composed of the nut of a tree, covered with what appears to be breadfruit resin. There are also traces of lime, which was used in the cleaning and caring of the skull. 18th century. Ex Christies London and formerly in the collections of Patricia Withoffs and Lord McAlpine, both of London.

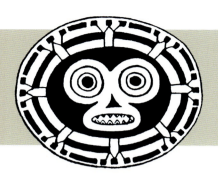

MARQUESAS

The Marquesas consist of ten substantial islands and a few minor islets. Lying approximately 2,000 miles southeast of Easter Island and 1,800 miles northeast of Tahiti, they are of ancient volcanic origin with a wide variety of dramatic terrain. On the islands of Ua Pou, Nuku Hiva and Hiva Oa, there are deep valleys rising to rugged central peaks, some reaching over 4,000 feet.

Because of the geological makeup of the islands, there are almost no areas of fringing coral reef, as the coastal cliffs descend to great depths. This phenomenon combined with the cool waters of the Peruvian current prevents the growth of coral polyps. Fishing thus was somewhat limited, with agriculture being the mainstay and the cultivation of crops occurring only on the valley floors. The primary foodstuff was the breadfruit, being pounded in a substance known as *poipoi*. The other staples of the Polynesian diet included coconuts, bananas, sugarcane and taro. Pigs were also consumed and were one of the many items introduced by the first Polynesian settlers.

There is little variation in temperature in the island group with the average being around 78 degrees Fahrenheit. Rainfall in the islands can vary greatly with over 100 inches annually in eastern parts of the islands, while western areas receive considerably less, often resulting in devastating droughts when there is no rain at all. Because of this weather phenomenon, the eastern areas are extremely lush in vegetation while the western areas can be inhospitable and arid.

Isolation of the Marquesas resulted in pre-settlement flora and fauna being limited, with only a dozen or so land birds extant and no mammals. With the arrival of Polynesian settlers the necessary food plants and animals were introduced to sustain these "valley societies."

As in all areas of Polynesia, there is great speculation as to where and when the first voyagers arrived in a particular island group. According to Dr. Yoshi Sinoto, a date of 300 AD has been given with the first people arriving from the islands of Samoa.[1] During this long period of occupation before European contact, hereditary tribal territories were established in the various valleys. These "valley societies" occurred primarily due to the geographic makeup of the islands, with communication by sea the most efficient mode of contact.

The first Europeans to sight the Marquesas were the Spanish expedition under the command of Alvaro Mendana de Neyra (1541-1595) who discovered the the

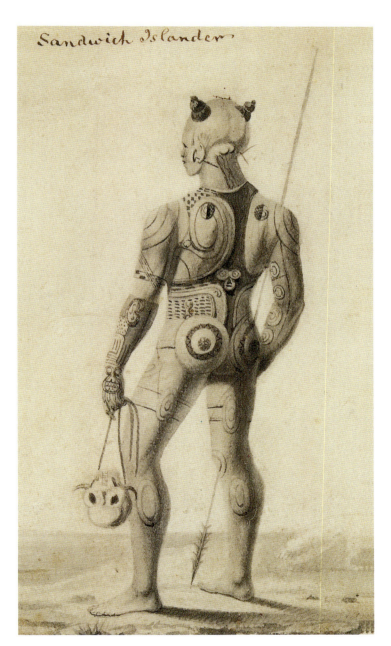

Original drawing entitled "Sandwich Islander." This small, mislabeled drawing is actually a drawing or a possible preparatory sketch of a Marquesan for an engraving from G.H. Von Langsdorff's Russian voyage of exploration published in 1813 in London. This sketch was found in an early album of calling cards from the late 18th and early 19th centuries that also contained, among other notable items, the calling card of the Tahitian Omai of Captain Cook's voyages, the first tattooed Polynesian to visit England.

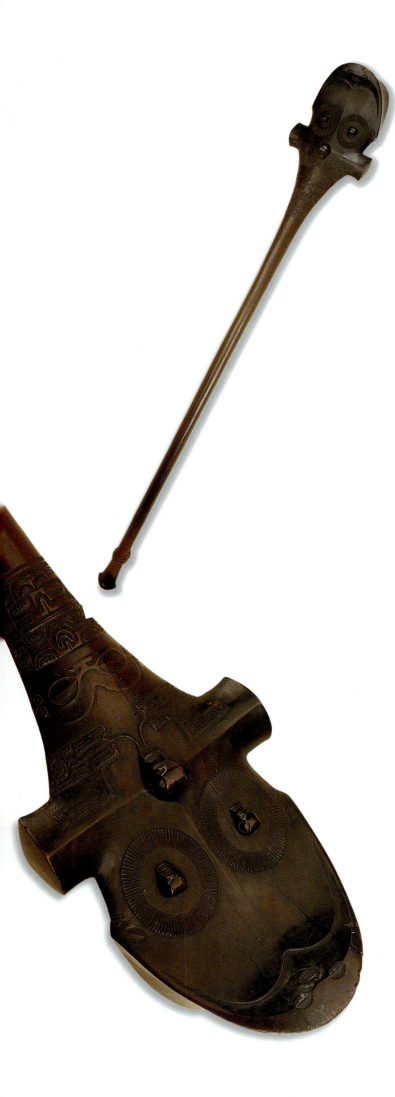

southern group in 1595.[2] This first encounter turned bloody at the end of their stay when several hundred Marquesans were slaughtered at the Bay of Virgins over a minor transgression.[3] The next European to appear was Captain James Cook who arrived for a short stay on his second voyage of discovery nearly two hundred years later in April 1774. It was on Cook's voyage that we have the first detailed reference to actual tattooing.[4]

> The Inhabitents of these Isles are without exception as fine a race of people as any in this Sea or perhaps any whatever; the Men are Tattowed or curiously Marked from head to foot like a coat of Mail which makes them look dark but the Women (who are but little Tattow'd) youths and children are as fair as some Europeans…

This, along with a comment by Forster recorded at Tahu Ata stating that the designs in the tattoo motifs are not naturalistic but geometric, taking the form of "blotches, spirals, bars, and chequers, and lines," is the only real reference from this brief contact.

After Cook's encounter, the French trading ship *Le Solide* arrived in the Marquesas under the command of Captain E. Marchand in 1791, stopping for a few days in the southern group. Upon sailing northwards, he discovered Ua Pou on June 21, having just missed the American trader Ingraham who encountered the rest of the group and proceeded to name them the Washington Islands in honor of the first president. Over the next fifty or so years there were numerous visits to the Marquesas by traders and official expeditions. Three Russian explorers, Krusenstern, Langsdorff, and Lisiansky were the first to illustrate tattooing in depth and provide lengthy ethnographic descriptions after visiting the islands at the be-

Marquesan *U'u* club. This superb club is carved from dense-grained *toa* wood and represents one of the crowning achievements in Marquesan woodcarving by the specialist woodworking *tuhuna*. Formidable weapons, these double-headed war clubs are without a doubt one of the most powerful and inventive objects in all of Polynesia. The massive club head is composed of two primary faces back to back, divided by a saddle-back ridge with a broad groove that can accommodate an arm pit, and were often used to lean on. The *U'u* club is a forceful sculptural form that masterfully incorporates minor sculptural elements along with exacting surface relief designs, many of them incorporating various motifs seen in Marquesan tattoo. Several stylized head or facial representations can be seen individually, all of which flow in harmony and balance on a single stylized head. After the club was completed at a high cost to the commissioner, it was finely sanded with sharkskin and placed in the mud of a taro patch for curing and blackening.* Afterwards, the club would be regularly rubbed and polished with scented coconut oil, which produced a glossy lacquer-like finish. Due to their high cost, clubs were limited to use by chiefs and other men of high rank, thus serving as symbols of prestige and items of formidable power in war. Clubs used to kill were given the commemorative names of their victims. Being highly valued and bequeathed as treasured heirlooms, they were coveted as potentially prized trophies in wars between opposing tribes. Height: 58-1/2 inches. 18th century.

*The blackening of these clubs may have had some correlation to the blackening of the skin in tattooing.

ginning of the 19th century. Their published accounts are some of the most invaluable that exist and provide elaborate illustrations of Marquesan tattoo art.

The islands provided a haven for all types of beachcombers who jumped ship in the late 18th and 19th centuries. It was the Frenchman Jean Baptiste Cabri who was the first recorded European to be tattooed in the Marquesas, obtaining traditional elaborate tattoos after jumping ship. In a journal kept by Edward Robarts,[5] another beachcomber at the time, Cabri is described as a madman. Cabri was well known for aggravating Robarts by interfering with European explorers and traders who passed through the islands. Cabri, after leaving the Marquesas some years later, made a living by travelling through Europe displaying his tattoos and entertaining groups with his romantic South Sea stories. After his death his skin was preserved and displayed - a rather gruesome legacy.

Marquesan society at the time of European contact was composed of large descent groups (*huaka*) confined to the most hospitable valleys, and it is from these that the various tribes developed. Each tribe occupied a single valley or, in the case of larger valleys, shared with other tribes. It was only on the island of Ua Pou that a single tribe controlled the entire island. The Marquesans were well known for their fighting ability, and warfare was frequent, causing expulsion from tribal lands. Most fighting, though, was limited to sporadic border skirmishes.

The tribes were held together by a chief, but his or her powers were not despotic and commoners were assured a reasonable sense of security with tenure of their plantations and family plots. Marquesan society was somewhat different from other areas of Polynesia. The position of the chief was not exclusively hereditary nor was the society rigidly stratified. Any person, male or female, could rise to this high rank as long as he was the first born (*hara-iki*). Marriage was as not as strictly regulated as in other Polynesian societies with genealogical status not playing such an important role with a child automatically taking on the rank of his senior parent. It was also in this society, unlike other areas in Polynesia, that women of humble birth were not seen as *mana*-polluting agents, as there were no low or depised classes.

The *mana* and *tapu* system was present but not as defined as in other island groups, although all first-born males were subject to some of these regulations by virtue of their genealogical position. Illness, famine, etc., were considered divine punishments for *tapu* transgressions.

Like other areas of Polynesia the four major gods were present: *Tu* the patron of war, *Tangaroa* responsible for the sea and winds, *Tane* and *Ono (Rongo)*, with the latter two being not so important as in other areas of Polynesia. One of the more famous gods in the Marquesan pantheon was *Tiki*, who was a demi-god of heroic nature appearing in numerous legends and stories. Gods intervened in everyday affairs, either directly or indirectly through inspirational priests (*tou'a*) whose capacity for spiritualness gave them considerable prestige. The class of priests known as *tuhuna o'ono* were the ones responsible for ritual and preservation of tribal lore. Rituals in the Marquesas took place in sacred areas of large stone-paved festival centers known as *tohua*, this area being preserved for communal tribal activity. In this sacred area known as *me'ae*, human sacrifices were occasionally offered to the gods through great ritual and circumstance, although not necessarily on a regular basis. Usually this was reserved for the securing of a good harvest, breaking of a drought or some other area of serious concern.

Large wood and stone *tiki*, some of immense size, were erected on the *me'ae* and, according to passed-down tradition, represented deified *tribal* ancestors who had been famous in their time and through whom spirits had become deities of the tribe.

Households were not concentrated in villages but near the families' plantations. The chiefs' houses tended to be the largest and were the center of the community, having the sacred *me'ae* adjacent along with the old men and warrior houses. Breadfruit, of which many varieties were cultivated, was the staple food and provided sustenance in time of famine when it was stored in paste form in leaf- and stoned-lined pits, sometimes for several years.

In 1842, the French Admiral Dupetit-Thouar (1793-1864) annexed the islands for France ensuring French control of the area. This was seen as an important move as France had seen the failure of their installation around Akaroa in New Zealand; with the Treaty of Waitangi, New Zealand was linked to England forever. It was during this decade that the American writer Herman Mellville romanced the world with his description of the Marquesas in his two books *Typee* and *Omoo* loosely based upon his stay in the islands in the same year as the French annexation.

The islanders continued to live in basic isolation, but in 1863 a terrible smallpox epidemic wiped out most of the population of the northern islands. In the next unfortunate chain of events the Catholic Church, through their innumerable persecutions, repressed the local population resulting in rebellion on the island of Hiva Oa in 1880.

Continuing their pattern of isolation, the world was again made aware of these islands when the famous artist Paul Gauguin moved to Atuona on the island of Hiva Oa in September 1901. There he was finally able to get closer to the primitive, unspoiled paradise for which he was so desperately searching. He continued to paint until his death on May 8, 1903. During this period he produced several masterworks reflecting his brilliant genius until the very end.

Due to their isolation in the middle of the Pacific and to their great distance from any continental landmass, the islands today - without a doubt - represent the last totally unspoiled area of Polynesia. Still under French administration, the islanders are seeking their total independence, but this may be impossible after years of subsidies paid to the population due to the French spin-off of nuclear colonialism.[6] Only time will tell if the islanders' fortitude and hard work will result in such a situation.

Marquesan Tattooing – *patiki*

Marquesan tattooing was the most complex of any tattooing in the Pacific or, for that manner, the world. Like most other areas in Polynesia it consisted of pricking the skin with a toothed tattooing comb carrying a dark vegetal pigment. Once the dye was under the skin it would remain in a permanent state creating a deep blue marking in a variety of complex and highly ornate designs.

Tattooing in the Marquesas was a highly ritualized art form. Like most areas in Polynesia, there were complex traditions and rituals involved in the process of tattooing. The tattoo artist or *tuhuna* was a highly skilled artisan who was well paid for his work in the form of war clubs, pigs, tapa or ornaments. Assistants and helpers would erect a special house for the lengthy and time-consuming process and always accompanied the *tuhuna*. Often it would take many years for the family to pay for the tattooing of their eldest son or *opou*.[7]

Tattoos usually were applied at the onset of puberty in both males and females marking their physical and social maturity. Ruling chiefs and warriors were the ones with the most elaborate tattoos according to early narratives describing the islands. Polynesian tattoo specialist Tricia Allen, of Honolulu, has noted that tattooed men and women were far more desirable in marriage. This was not because they were more attractive in their prospective mate's eyes, but because tattooing indicated both strength and status and was considered a sign of wealth and endurance.[8] It also appears that the full-body tattoo acted as a type of armor prior to and up to the onset of European weaponry.

In one of the most remarkable descriptions of tattooing in Polynesia, G.H. Von Langsdorff describes what he saw in the Marquesas during his official Russian voyage of discovery around the world in the years 1803-1807:

> Among all the known nations of earth, none have carried the art of tattooing to so high a degree of perfection as the inhabitants of the Washington Islands. The regular designs with which the bodies of the men of Nukahiwa are punctured from head to foot supplies in some sort the absence of clothing; for, under so warm a heaven, clothing would be insupportable to them. Many people here seek as much to obtain distinction by the symmetry and regularity with which they are tattooed, as among us by the elegant manner in which they are dressed; and although no real elevation of rank is designated by the greater superiority of these decorations, yet as only persons of rank can afford to be at expence attendant upon any refinement in the ornaments, it does become in fact a badge of distinction.
>
> The operation is performed by certain persons, who gain their livelihood by it entirely, and I presume that those who perform it with the greatest dexterity, and evince the greatest degree of taste in the disposition of the ornaments, are as much sought after as among us a particularly good tailor. Thus much, however, must be said, that the choice made is not a matter of equal indifference with them as with us; for if the punctured garment be spoiled in the making, the mischief is irreparable, it must be worn with all its faults the whole life through.
>
> For performing the operation, the artist uses the wing bone of a tropic bird (*phaeton aethereus*) which is jagged and pointed at the end after the manner of a comb, sometimes in the form of a crescent, sometimes in a strait line, and larger or smaller according to the figures which the artist intends to make. This instrument is fixed into a bamboo handle about as thick as the finger, with which the puncturer, by means of another cane, strikes so gently and dexterously, that it scarcely pierces through the skin. The principle strokes of the figures to be tattooed are first sketched upon the body with the same dye that is afterwards rubbed into the punctures, to serve as guides in the use of the instrument. The punctures being made so that the blood and lymph ooze through the

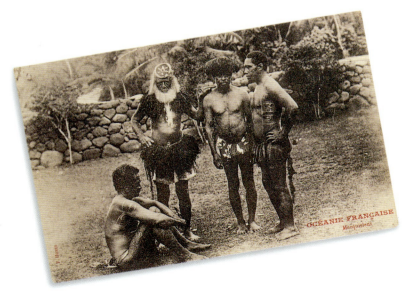

"Four Marquesan Types." A wonderful "staged" photo showing Marquesan men with traditional tattoos and garb. Original postcard published by Frank Homes* circa 1915.
*Frank Homes (1868-1953) was another of Tahiti's premier photographers documenting all of French Polynesia through a series of photographic prints and postcards and was closely linked with the Spitz enterprises. A jeweler by trade, he arrived in Tahiti in 1888 and married Alice Gooding, an heiress of much wealth. She owned a tremendous amount of land throughout the islands of French Polynesia.

orifice, a thick dye, composed of ashes from the kernel of the burning-nut (*aleurites triloba*) mixed with water, is rubbed in. This occasions at first a slight degree of smarting and inflammation, it then heals, and when the crust comes off, after some days the bluish or blackish-blue figure appears.

As soon as the inhabitant of Nukahiwa approaches towards the age of manhood, the operation of tattooing is begun, and this is one of the most important epochs of his life. The artist is sent for, and the agreement made with him that he is to receive so many hogs as his pay; the number is commonly regulated according to the wealth of the person to be tattooed, and the quantity of decoration bestowed is regulated by the pay. While we were at the island, a son of the chief Katanuah was to be tattooed. For this purpose, as belonging to the principal person in the island, he was put into a separate house for several weeks which was tabooed; that is to say, it was forbidden to everybody, except those who were exempted from taboo by his father, to approach the house; here he was to remain during the whole time that the operation continued. All women, even the mother, are prohibited from seeing the youth while the taboo remains in force. Both the operator and the operatee are fed with the very best food during the continuance of the operation: to the former these are the days of great festivity. In the first year only the ground-work of the principal figures upon the breast, arms, back, and thighs, is laid; and in doing this, the first punctures must be entirely healed, and the crust must have come off before new ones are to heal; and the first sitting, as it may be called, commonly lasts three or four weeks.

While the patient is going through the operation, he must drink very little, for fear of creating too much inflimation, and he is not allowed to eat early morning, only at noon and in the evening. When once the decorations are begun, some addition is constantly made to them at intervals of from three to six months, and this is not unfrequently continued for thirty or forty years before the whole tattooing is completed. We saw some old men of the higher ranks, who were punctured over and over to such a degree, that the outlines of each separate figure were scarcely to be distinguished, and the body had almost negro-like appearance. This is, according to the general idea, the height of perfection in ornament, probably because the cost of it has been very great, and it therefore shews a person of superlative wealth. It is singular, that the men of distinction should place their gratification in acquiring this dark hue, while the women place theirs in preserving their original fair complexion uninjured.

The tattooing of persons in a middling station is performed in houses erected for the purpose by tattooers, and tabooed by authority. A tattooer, who visited us several times on board the ship, had three of these houses, which could each receive eight or ten persons at a time: they paid for their decorations according to the greater or less quanity of them, and to the trouble the figures required. The poorer islanders, who have not a superabundance of hogs to dispose of in luxuries, but live chiefly themselves upon bread-fruit, are operated upon by novices in the art, who take them at a very low price as subjects of practice, but their works are easily distinguishable, even by a stranger, from those of an experienced artist. The lowest class of all, the fishermen principally, but few of whom we saw, are often not able to afford even the pay required by a novice, and are therefore not tattooed at all.

The women of Nukahiwa are very little tattooed, differing in this respect from the females of the other South-Sea islands. The hands are punctured from the ends of the fingers to the wrist, which gives them the appearance of wearing gloves, and our glovers might very well borrow from them patterns, and introduce a new fashion among ladies, of gloves worked "a la Washington". The feet, which among many are tattooed, look like highly-ornamented half-boots; long stripes are besides sometimes to be seen down the arms of the women, and circles round them, which have much the same effect as the bracelets worn by European ladies. Some also have their ears and lips tattooed. The women are not, like the men, shut up in a tabooed house while they are going through this operation: it is performed without any ceremony in their own houses, or in those of their relations: in short, wherever they please.

Sometimes a rich islander will, either from generosity, ostentation, or love to his wife, make a feast in honour of her, when she has a bracelet tattooed round her arm, or perhaps her ear ornamented; a hog is then killed, and the friends of both sexes are invited to partake of it, the occasion of the feast being made known to them. It is expected that the same courtesy should be returned in case of the wife of any of the guests being punctured. This is one of the few occasions women are allowed to eat hog's flesh. If, in a very dry year, bread-fruit, hogs, roots, and other provisions become scarce, anyone who has still a good stock of them, which commonly happens to the chief, in order to distribute his stores, keeps open table for a certain time to an appointed number of poor artists, who are bound to give in return some strokes of the tattoo to all who choose to come for it. By virtue of a taboo, all these bretheren are engaged to support each other, if in future some happen to be in need, while the others are in affluence. This is one of the most rational orders of Free-masonry upon the globe.

Our interpreter Cabri, who was slightly and irregularly tattooed all over his body, upon one of these occasions got a black, or rather blue eye; and Roberts, who had only a puncture on his breast, in the form of a long square, six inches one way and four the other, assured us that that he would never have submitted to the operation, if he had not been constrained by the scarcity the preceeding year to become one of the guests fed by the chief Katanuah. The same person may be a member of several of these societies; but, according to what we could learn, a portion must always be given to the priest or magician, as he is called, even if he be not a member. In a time of scarcity also, many of the people who have been tattooed in this way unite as an absolute troop of banditti, and share equally among each other all they can plunder and kill.

The figures with which the body is tattooed are chosen with great care, and appropriate ornaments are selected for the different parts. They consist partly of animals, partly of other objects which have some reference to the manners and customs of the islands; and every figure has here, as in the Friendly Islands, its particular name. Upon an accurate examination, curved lines, diamonds, and other designs, are often distinguishable between rows of punctures, which resemble very much the ornaments "a la Grecque". The most perfect symmetry is observed over the whole body: the head of a man is tattooed in every part; the breast is commonly ornamented with a figure resembling a shield; on the arms and thighs are stripes, sometimes broader, sometimes narrower, in such directions that these people might very well be presumed to have studied anatomy, and to be aquainted with the course and dimensions of the muscles. Upon the back is a large cross, which begins at the neck, and ends with the last vertabrae. In the front of the thigh are often figures, which seem intended to represent the human face. On each side the calf of the leg is an oval figure, which produces a very good effect. The whole, in short, displays much taste and discrimination. Some of the tenderest parts of the body, the eye-lids for example, are the only parts not tattooed."[9]

The French eventually outlawed tattooing in the Marquesas in 1884 because of the lobbied efforts of the Catholic Church. Noted writer Robert Louis Stevenson's mother, in her book of letters *From Saranac to the Marquesas*, recorded what appeared to be fairly recent tattooing on women on the island of Nuku Hiva in 1888:

> They wore light-coloured holakus with long trains, a very pretty garment, in which they looked most graceful; their feet were bare, but tattooed in such beautiful patterns that they had the appearance of wearing open-work silk stockings. They tattoo their legs all over, and Fanny and I feel very naked with our own plain white legs when we are bathing."[10]

This passage illustrates the great sense of beauty and awe that many visitors felt when they encountered tattooing in the Marquesas.

Design elements were very numerous as described in the above early firsthand accounts. In Willowdean Handy's bulletin from the Bishop Museum's Bayard Dominick Expedition[11] to the Marquesas in 1921, she observed tattoos on 125 persons. It was her conclusion, after many discussions with her informants, that there were various reasons for covering different parts of the body with tattoo. In some of her more important findings based upon the informants, she was told that the decorated hand was noticeable in kneading and eating *poipoi*. The underarm patterns made a fine showing and distracted the opponent when the arms were uplifted in striking with a war club. Shoulder and chest decorations were displayed when a man walked with arms crossed behind his back. It was also said that the circular motifs on the inside of the knees were in evidence and much admired when men sat cross-legged and that the insides of the thighs were deliberately left vacant as they were covered by loin cloths.

There is much speculation as to whether certain design elements, especially on the face, designated tribal markings. In an early reference, Porter makes a statement to this effect but it cannot be substantiated in any other source.[12] Many tattoo design elements were recorded during the 18th and 19th centuries – even Herman Mellville stated in 1843 that he saw fish, birds, and trees tattooed on natives of Nuku Hiva. In addition to the naturalistic motifs, geometric motifs also were recorded.

Many of these motifs are found in classic Marquesan woodcarving as is illustrated here in these pages. Whether the design elements first appeared as woodcarving and decoration is anyone's guess. This along with the standardizing of design elements by island areas is another area of debate. Willowdean Handy made a strong case in her Bishop Museum Bulletin:

> An examination of the extant examples of the art shows a distinct cleavage between the two groups in their conception of design, that of the southeastern group being purely conventional with but minor relics of the geometric and the slightest trace of the naturalistic art, many of the geometric, and a simpler form of the conventional than the other. Marquesans are all agreed, that, as far as tattooing customs went, the islands were divided into two groups: Nuku Hiva and Ua Pou forming one; Hiva Oa, Tahu Ata, Fatu Hiva and Ua Huka – because of its close intercourse with the north and west coast of Hiva Oa forming the other.

She further states Hiva Oa was considered to be the center for all the tattoo arts.

Today there is a new awakening of the art of tattoo in the Marquesas. On a trip made to all the islands in the early 1990s, the author saw many examples of tattooing, but this was mainly limited to males who worked on copra ships that plied their trade back and forth between the islands and Tahiti. In Tahiti today it is very stylish to have tattoos in Marquesan designs applied. Design elements from Marquesan tattooing are seen throughout French Polynesia, in commercial forms including advertising, business logos, clothing designs, and even architectural elements – all a rather odd tribute to the tattoo artists of the past.

TRANSLATION OF NAMES ACCORDING TO HANDY

aa fanaua	row of evil spirits
akaaka fa'a	pandanus roots
enata	man
fa'a mana	pandanus branches
fanaua	a kind of evil spirit
fatina	jointure
hei ta'avaha	a diadem of cock's plumes
hei po'i'i	shellfish or wreath
hikuhiku atu	bonito fish tails
honu	turtle
hue ao	calabash bottom
hue epo	dirty calabash
hue tai	compass
ihu epo	dirty nose
ikeike	a kind of shrub
ipu ani	sky bowl
ipu ao	bowl bottom
ipu oto	inside the bowl
iti'iti'i	binding
ka'ake	armpit
ka'ava	ridge pole
kaka'a	lizard
kea	woodlouse, turtle or carved turtle shell plaque
kikipu	lips
kikomata	eyes
kikutu	lips
kohe ta	sword
kohe tua	back knife
kopiko	zigzag
koua'ehi	coconut leaves
makamaka	branches
mata	eyes
mata hoata	brilliant eye
niho	teeth
nihoniho peata	shark teeth
nutu kaha	mouth
omuo puaina	carved bone earring
pahito	ancient patch
paka	splinter
paka oto	inside places
pakiei	crab
pana'o	cut in small slices
papua	enclosure or garden
papua au ti	enclosure of ti leaves
papua enata	native enclosure
peata	shark
peka tua	back cross
peke ou mei	a kind of evil spirit
pia'o tiu	to fold or bundle
Pohu	a legendary figure
po'i'i'	a coiled shellfish
poka'a	wooden shoulder rest for a carrying pole
pu	conch shell
puaina, puainga	ear
pua hitu	flower of olden times
pua hue	flower calabash
puha puaka	pig's thigh
puto'o	buttocks
tamau	ring
tapu vae	sacred foot
ti'ati'a pu	to encircle several times
tifa	cover
tiki	image
tiki ae	forehead image
tou pae	three head ornaments
tumu ima	hand tree
vahana ae	half a forehead
vai me'ama	water moon
vai o Kena	water of Kena, a legendary hero
vai ta keetu	sacred bathing place of chiefs
veo	tail
vi'i po'i'i	to turn the shell fish

Endnotes

[1] Yoshi Sinoto from Bishop Museum in Honolulu has done extensive field work in the Marquesas and has suggested this "settlement phase" although challenging some of the most recent radiocarbon dating that could bring the date back to as early as 200 BC.

[2] The islands thus were named Las Marquesas de Mendoca, in honor of the Marquis de Canete, governor of Peru, who had been given charge of overseeing the expedition. The expedition's chief mission was to find gold in the Solomon Islands.

[3] One of Mendana's soldiers admitted killing a nursing mother to prove his prowess as a good shot, with his camp master stating: "because to kill is our pleasure and profession…and what matter if the heathen are consigned to hell today since they will go there in any case tomorrow?"

[4] Quiros, the pilot of Mendana's voyage in 1595, recorded in his journal during their visit to the southeastern islands the observation of "fish and other patterns painted" upon the faces and bodies of natives.

[5] *The Marquesan Journal of Edward Roberts*, G.M. Dening (ed.), Canberra, Australia, 1974.

[6] The French nuclear testing at Muraroa in the Tuamotu Islands brought in large subsidies of monies in all areas of French Polynesia including the Marquesas. Without these subsidies that the islanders have been so dependent on for several decades, it may be difficult for them to become self-sufficient. The only export item of any means is copra, which has seen its price depressed over the last several years. Tourism is virtually non-existent.

[7] An *opou* was the eldest son of a wealthy family.

[8] This according to her booklet entitled *European Explorers and Marquesan Tattooing - The Wildest Island Style*, Handy Marks Publication, Honolulu, 1990.

[9] This important description of tattooing has been added in its entirety due to its highly accurate and remarkable description of Marquesan culture at a time when traditional ways of life were basically still intact.

[10] *From Saranac to the Marquesas and Beyond - being letters written by Mrs. M. I. Stevenson during 1887-1888, to her sister Jane Whyte Balfour*. Edited and arranged by Marie Clothilde Balfour, Methuen and Co., London, 1903.

[11] This officially sanctioned expedition by the Bishop Museum of Honolulu was invaluable in recording many aspects of Marquesan culture. It was published in various bulletins by the museum. The tattoo bulletin was Number One published in 1922.

[12] *Journal of a Voyage to the Pacific Ocean in the United States Frigate* Essex *in the year 1812-1814*, two volumes, Philadelphia, 1815.

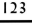

Original watercolor of a Marquesan warrior. In this contemporary picture by one of Tahiti's most famous artists, Jean-Louis Saquet, an engraving from the voyage of the *Le Breton* in 1838 under the command of Admiral Dumont d' Urville* has been used for inspiration. This dramatic picture illustrates both the beauty and power of traditional Marquesan tattooing.
*Admiral Dumont d' Urville commanded a French scientific expedition that anchored for about a week in Nuka Hiva. From this voyage were published numerous engravings along with a written account by Vincendon Dumoulin.

Right: Original photograph of a Marquesan man. A wonderful "staged" studio portrait by Frank Homes circa 1900. This is the same person as is illustrated on page 140, but in this albumen photograph he is wearing a variety of traditional objects including a rare head ornament or *uhikana* carved from pearl and turtle shell on a woven coconut fiber band. He is wearing shoulder and wrist ornaments or *Motutu ovoho* of woven human hair. His hand is resting on a *U'u* club, a late example made for the curio market.

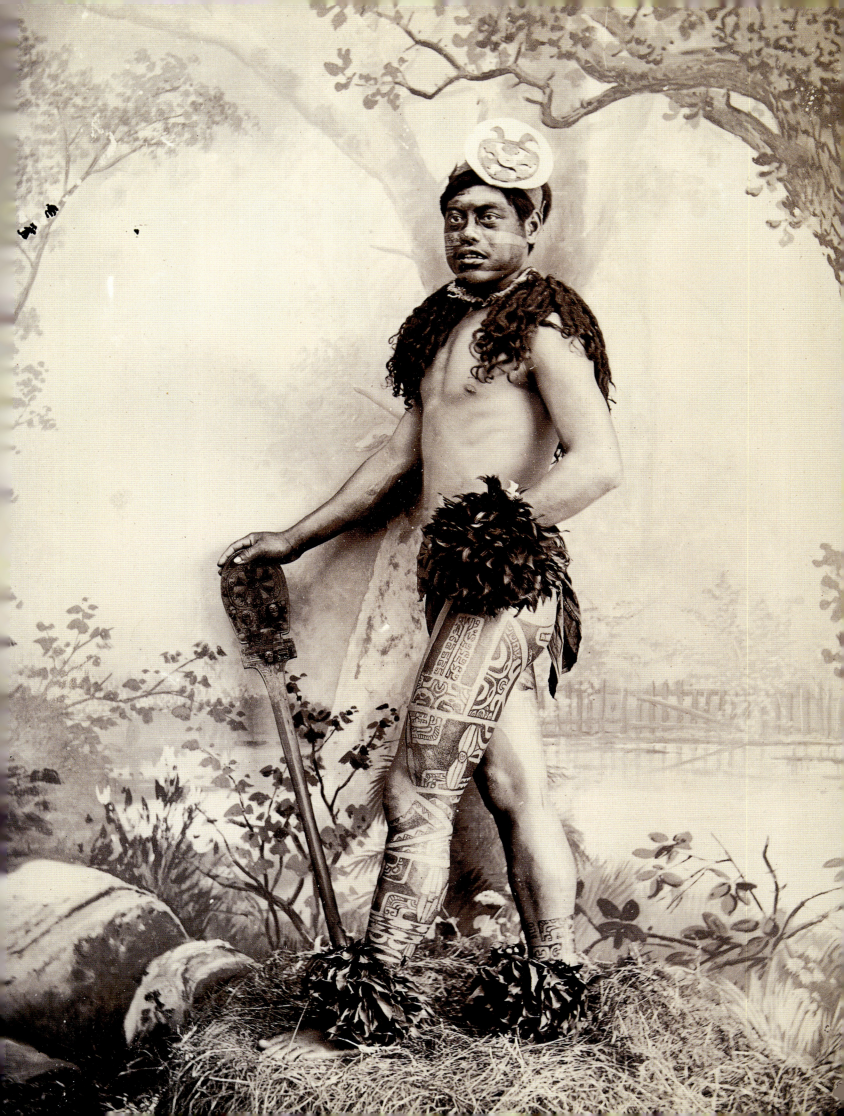

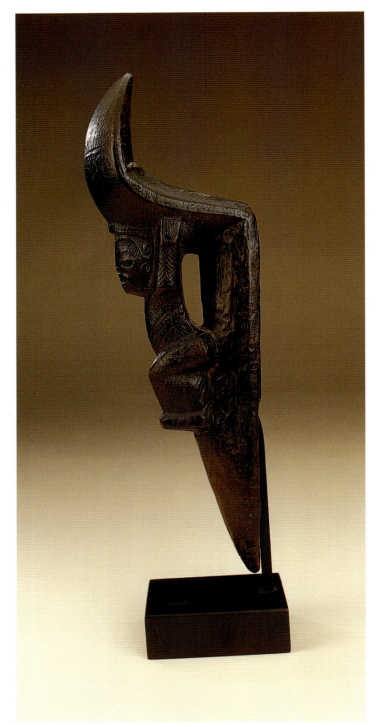
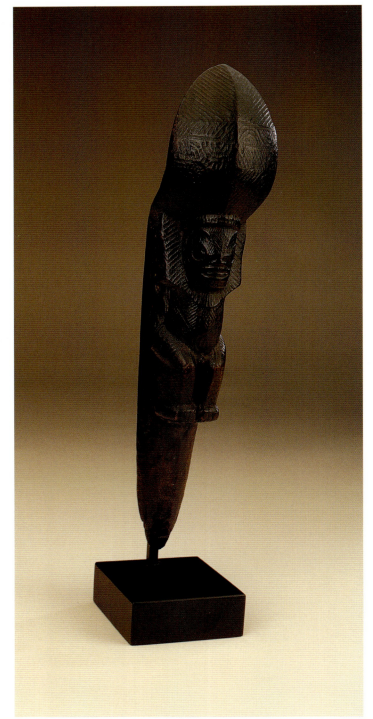

Marquesan stilt step *Tapuva'e*. Stilt walking and other contests of skill were favorite entertainment in the Marquesas Islands. Stilt poles were generally six feet in height, around two inches in diameter, and were constructed primarily of bamboo. Early accounts suggest that these poles were wrapped in white tapa with the figurative steps bound to the poles with ornamental lashings of red or black coconut fiber sennit. Formal contests were held during commemorative festivals where champions from various tribes competed against each other with wagering done by the various observers. In these contests each performer tried to force his opponent to the ground with well-practiced tripping maneuvers and defensive counter-measures. Accomplished stilt-walkers could perform somersaults and other acrobatic maneuvers while on stilts. These formal events were held on the paved stone enclosures of the *me'ae*, while less formal events and practicing were held in the village grounds. Like the *U'u* clubs, great care was taken in carving these stilts by the specialist woodworking *tuhuna*, with the final finishing process similar to clubs involving curing in the mud of a taro patch. Of great dynamic sculptural quality and always involving a centralized *tiki* form, they are often decorated as in this example, in tattoo-like motifs. This stilt is one of a pair purchased from the famous Marquesan collector Emil Bouchard in Paris and is unusual with its upraised arms. Height: 12-3/4 inches. 18th century.

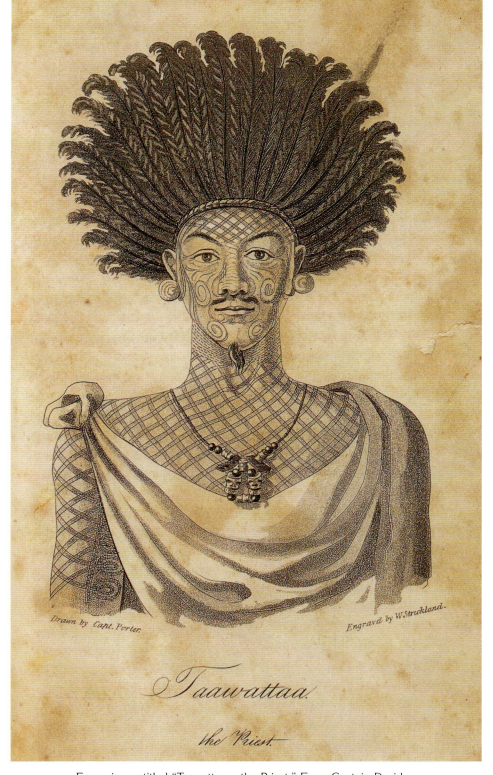

Engraving entitled "Taawattaa – the Priest." From Captain David Porter's *Journal of a Cruise made to the Pacific Ocean in the United States Frigate "Essex" in the years 1812-1814* and published in two volumes in Philadelphia in 1822. In this illustration the priest is shown with crosshatch pattern on his body, which may or may not be what Capt. Porter saw as Porter and the engraver may have used an immense amount of artistic license.

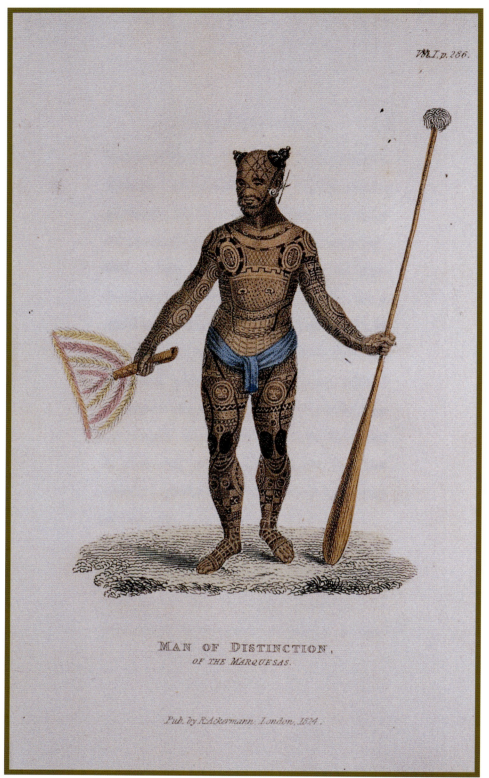

Engraving entitled "Man of Distinction, of the Marquesas." From *The World in Miniature – South Sea Islands*, published in 1824 in London, Frederick Shorbel editor. This handsome print is a rather fanciful depiction of Marquesan tattoo on a man of high rank.

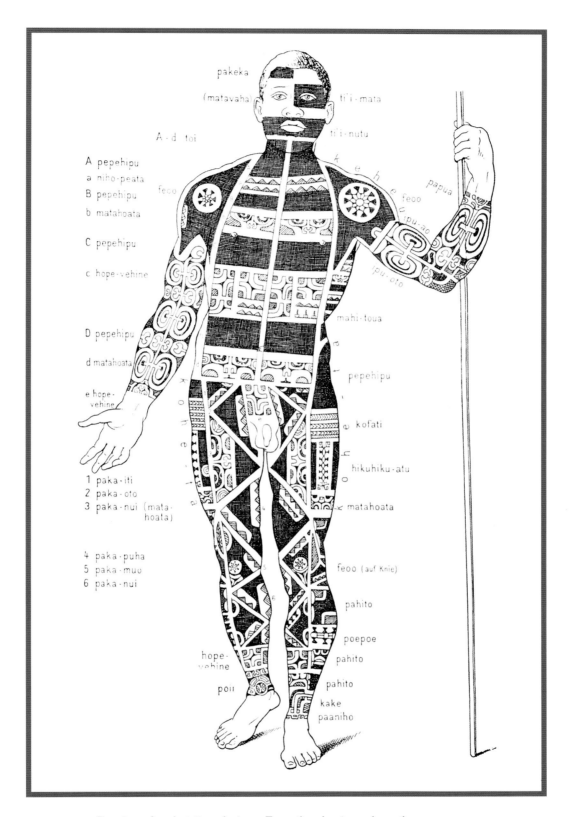

Drawing of male tattoo designs. From the classic work on the Marquesas by Karl von den Steinen *Die Marquesaner und ihre Kunst*,* published in Germany in 1925. A detailed drawing with accompanying Marquesan names showing design elements on a man of Hiva Oa.
*Karl von den Steinen's book, a classic on the Marquesan culture, was based upon his observances in the islands when he visited there as part of an official expedition sent by Berlin Ethnographic museum in 1897. Published as a three-volume set, it is an invaluable work, although many scholars criticize many of his interpretations of the people and the arts and culture he observed. He also collected many Marquesan myths at this time, these later being published in German. These myths are important in their relationships to designs on artifacts and tattoos, which often have legendary references.

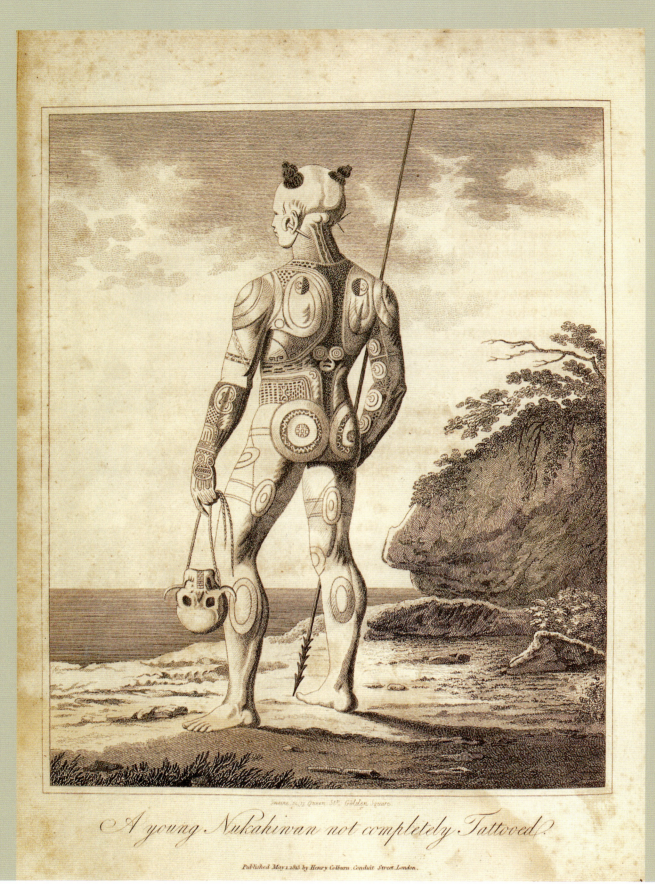

Engraving entitled "A young Nukahivan, not completely Tattooed." From G.H. Von Langsdorff's Russian voyage of exploration published in 1813 in London. This remarkable image is a good representation of partial back and leg tattoos. Complete body tattoos took many years of work and represented a tremendous amount of spent wealth and personal bravery, all due to the pain one had to incur in obtaining them, thus tattoos had associations with wealth and the ability to endure great pain. In his left hand this warrior is carrying a "trophy skull" of a powerful enemy. These were often carried into battle attached to the waist. The skulls, being heads, represent the most sacred part of the body and are imbued with *mana,* thus protecting the warrior in battle.

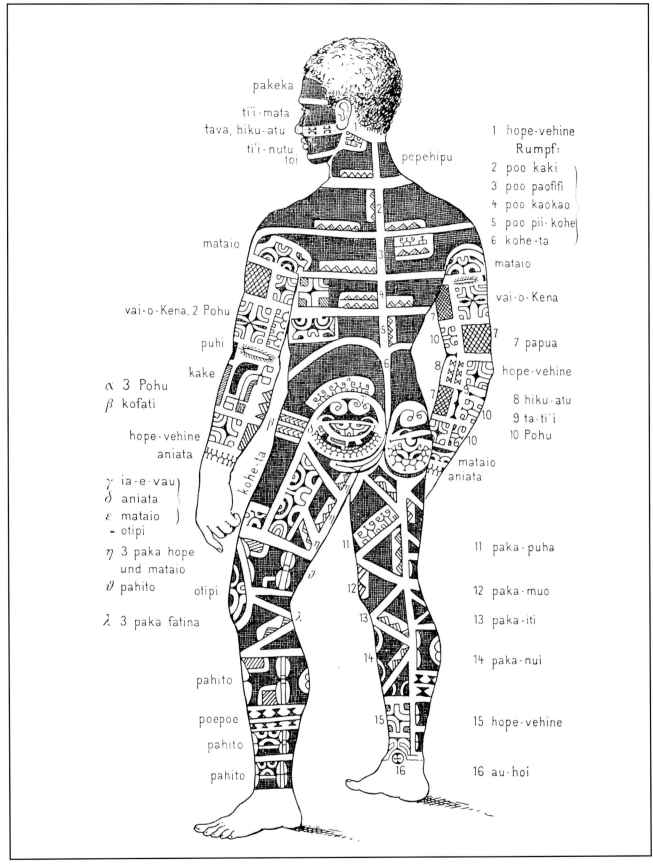

Drawing of male tattoo designs. From the classic work on the Marquesas by Karl von den Steinen *Die Marquesaner und ihre Kunst*, published in Germany in 1925. A detailed drawing with accompanying Marquesan names showing design elements on a *tahuna* of Hiva Oa.

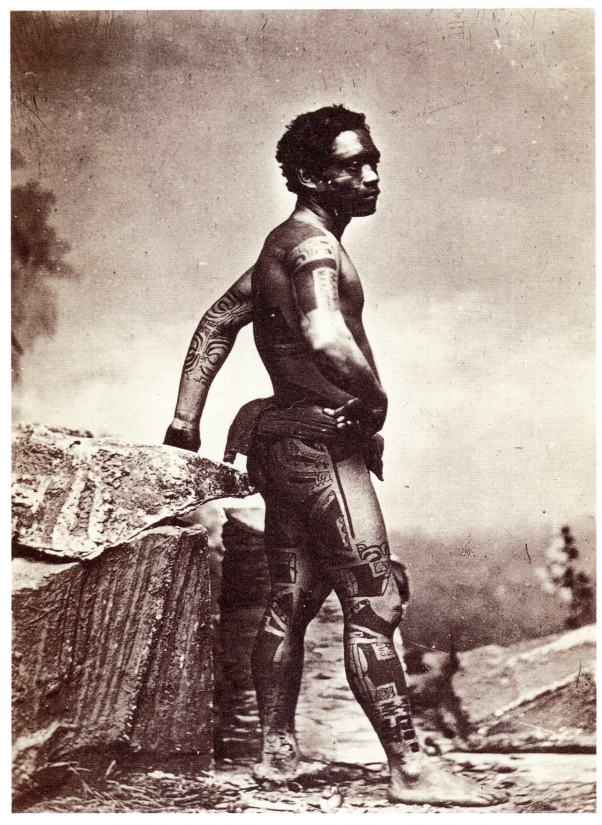

Original photograph of a Marquesan warrior. This interesting and rare photo shows a very good depiction of traditional tattooing as well as an unusual arm tattoo with what appears to be two words. Whether this is a memorial tattoo or the person's baptismal tattoo or some type of tattoo graffiti is not known. Original albumen photograph by Charles Spitz* circa 1880s.

*Charles Spitz (1857-1894) was one of Tahiti's premier photographers. He marketed his images through his Spitz Curio Store located in Papeete, which specialized in all sorts of South Sea curiosities. The firm was active for many years even after his death when his sons took over. All the original glass negatives were unfortunately lost in a hurricane except for a small number that are currently in the Blackburn Collection.

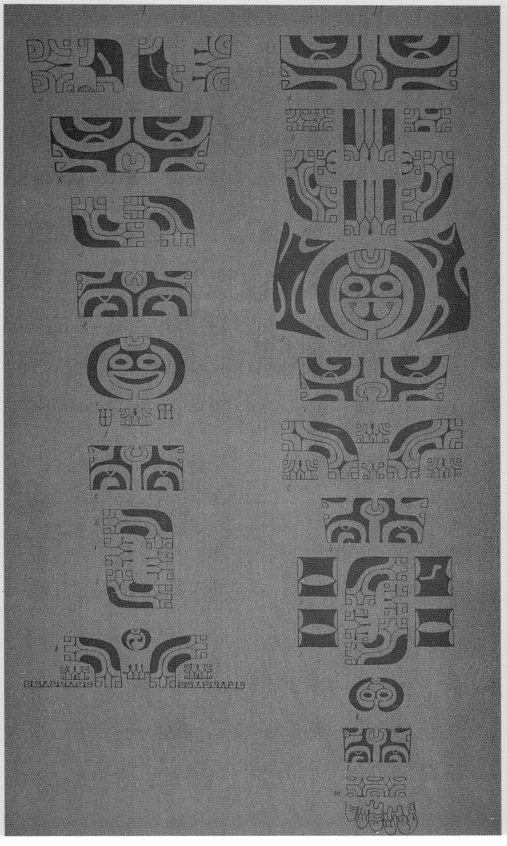

Color plate entitled "Tattoo Designs in the Marquesas." From Willowdean Chatterson Handy's* classic account published by Bishop Museum in 1921 entitled *Tattooing in the Marquesas*. This illustration is quite important as it shows the actual color as it appears on the skin. The design motifs are what Handy has labeled as a "modern type," indicating that in some isolated areas tattooing was still being done and was more degenerate in style. The designs in this plate are all leg patterns for women with their Marquesan names as collected by Handy as follows:

A. Back Pattern: *vai pahu* (a, left) *ka'ake* (a, center) *mata hoata* (b) *ka'ake* (c) *mata hoata* (d) *ipu ani* (e) *vai o Kena* (f) *mata hoata* (g) *ka'ake* (h) and (j) *Pohu* (i) *ipu ani* (k, center) *ka'ake* (k, left and right).

B. Front Pattern: *mata hoata* (a) *po'okohe* (b, left and right) *kea* (b, center) *ka'ake* (c, left and right) *pahito* (d, left and right) *ipu ani* (d, center) *mata mei nei* (e) *ka'ake* (f, left and right) *vai o Kena*, sometimes called *potia hue* or *peke ou mei* (f, center) *Pohu* (g, center) *mata hoata* (h) *pahito* (i and j, left and right) *ka'ake* (i and j, center) *ipu ani* (k) *mata hoata* (l) *etua poou*, sometimes *Pohu* (m).

*Willowdean Chatterson Handy served as a volunteer with Bishop Museum's Bayard Dominick Expedition to the Marquesas in 1920-1921. She kept an intimate record of tattooing designs that she encountered while on the expedition. At the time of her visit there were approximately 125 Marquesan people still wearing tattoos in the islands. Her attributions and studies are based upon what she observed during her stay, and with interviews conducted with her Marquesan informants. Her accuracy and interpretation are subject to considerable debate among scholars today.

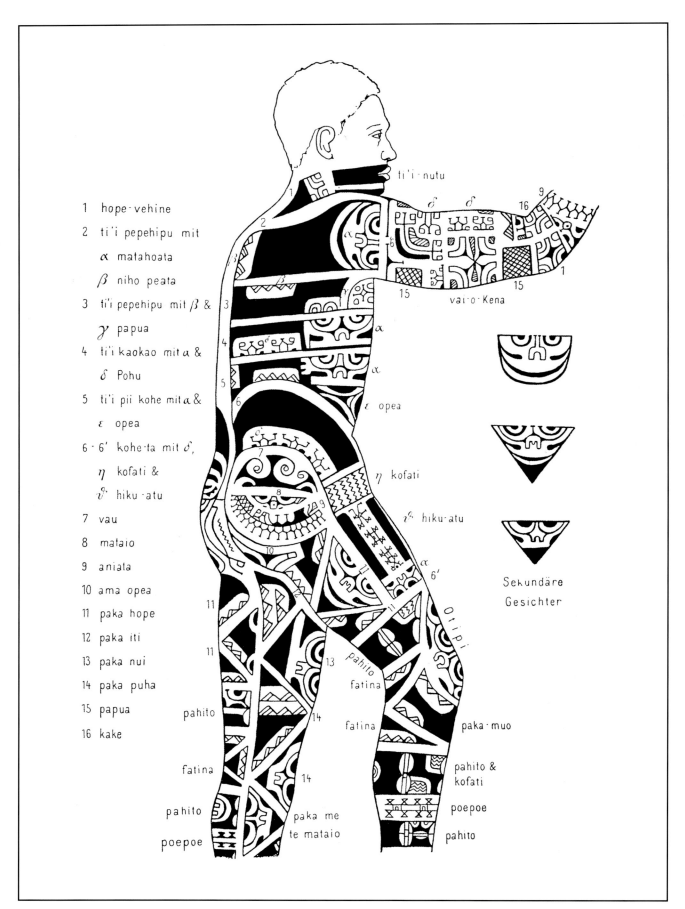

Drawing of male tattoo designs. From the classic work on the Marquesas by Karl von den Steinen *Die Marquesaner und ihre Kunst*, published in Germany in 1925. A detailed drawing with accompanying Marquesan names showing design elements on a *tahuna* of Hiva Oa.

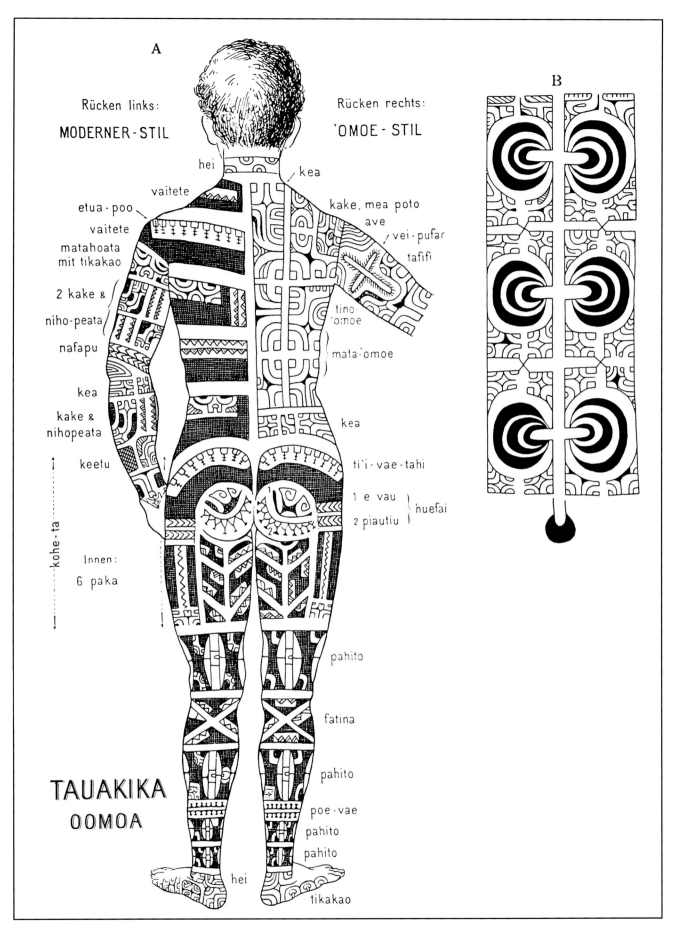

Drawing of male tattoo designs. From the classic work on the Marquesas by Karl von den Steinen *Die Marquesaner und ihre Kunst*, published in Germany in 1925. The detailed line drawing labeled A shows what he has described as the more modern style on the left and the traditional older style on the right. The Marquesan words recorded at the time of his visit for each design element are located next to the appropriate area. The drawing labeled B is of the inner and front sides of the arms. These drawings are based upon a composite of tattoos he saw in the Marquesas in 1897.

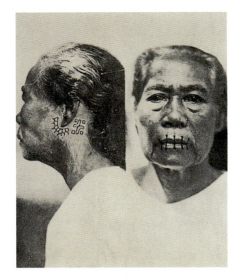

Photographs entitled "Tattoo Designs in the Marquesas." From Willowdean Chatterson Handy's classic account published by Bishop Museum in 1921 entitled *Tattooing in the Marquesas*. The top photograph shows lip and ear patterns, while the bottom photo shows frontal and rear views of the legs on the same woman whose name was Tuuakena from Atu Ona on the island of Hiva Oa.

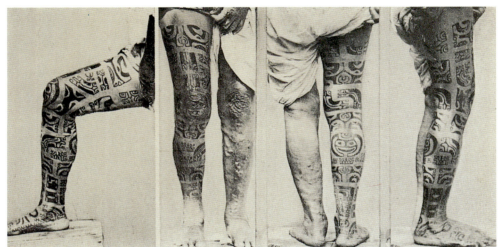

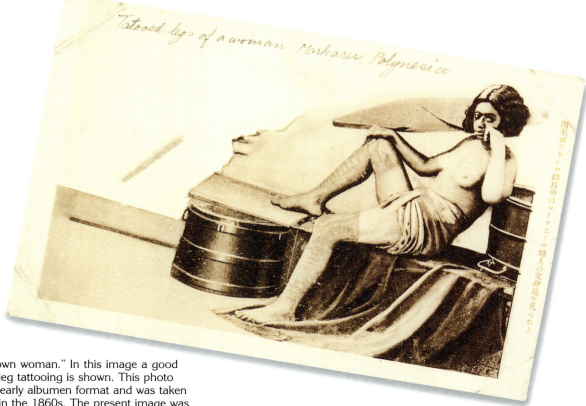

"Photograph of an unknown woman." In this image a good representation of female leg tattooing is shown. This photo originally appeared in an early albumen format and was taken aboard a ship sometime in the 1860s. The present image was lifted by a Japanese postcard publisher in the 1920s and was part of a series of "exotic peoples."

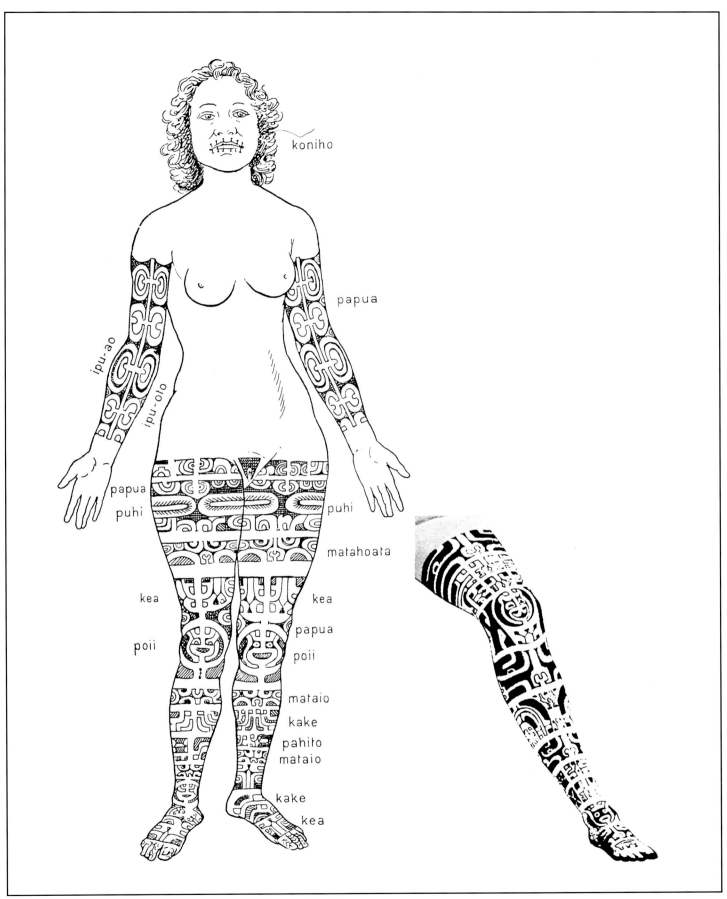

Drawing of female tattoo designs. From the classic work on the Marquesas by Karl von den Steinen *Die Marquesaner und ihre Kunst*, published in Germany in 1925. A detailed drawing with accompanying Marquesan names showing design elements on a woman from Hiva Oa.

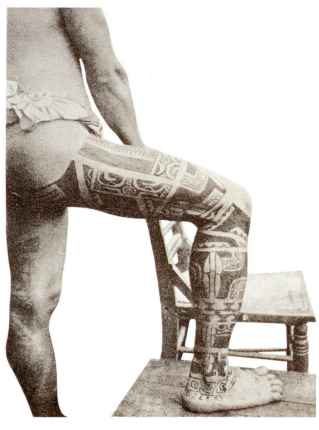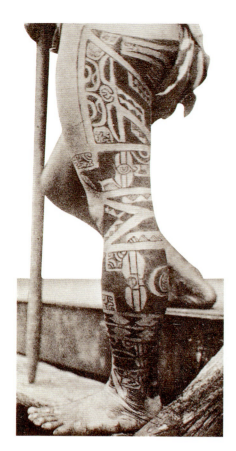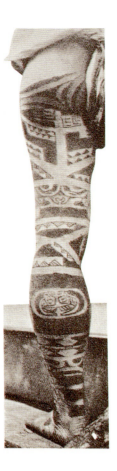

Above: Photograph of a man's legs, with side and back views. From the classic work on the Marquesas by Karl von den Steinen *Die Marquesaner und ihre Kunst*, published in Germany in 1925. This series of photographs shows various views of a leg from a man of Hiva Oa.

Below: Photograph entitled "Tattoo designs in the Marquesas." From Willowdean Chatterson Handy's classic account published by Bishop Museum in 1921 entitled *Tattooing in the Marquesas*. In this photograph Eotafa of Ta'a Oa of Hiva Oa is shown. Handy described this person as the most fully tattooed man in the Marquesas at the time. She added black paint to enhance the tattoo designs – she notes that identical patterns are on the unpainted half and do not appear in this photograph.

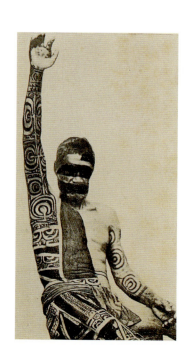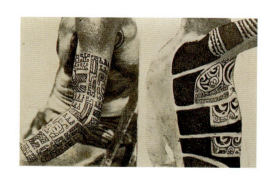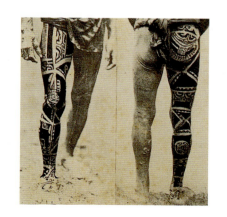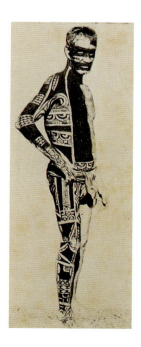

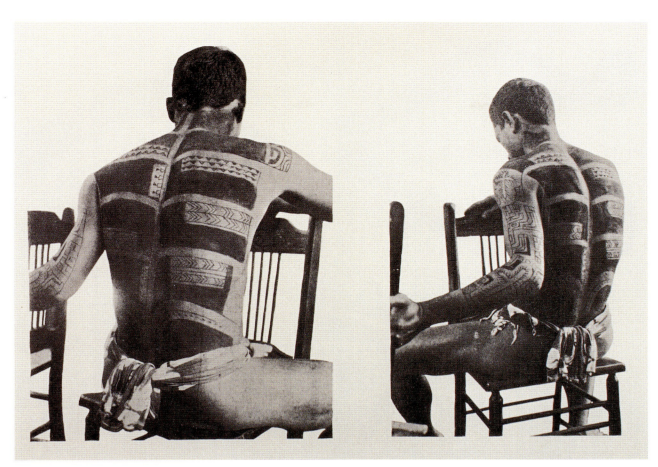

Above: Photographs showing two back views of a man. From the classic work on the Marquesas by Karl von den Steinen *Die Marquesaner und ihre Kunst*, published in Germany in 1925. These photos shows strong bold design elements featuring large areas of negative space. This man was photographed on the island of Hiva Oa in 1897.

Below: Photographs showing two back views of a man. From the classic work on the Marquesas by Karl von den Steinen *Die Marquesaner und ihre Kunst*, published in Germany in 1925. These photographs show back and detailed buttock tattoos of a man observed on the island of Hiva Oa. His body is only partially tattooed showing that he has many years of pain and courage to endure if he is to obtain a full-body tattoo. It is highly improbable that he ever obtained such a full-body tattoo as these photos were taken at a very late date in 1897 when traditional tattooing had been in decline for a number of years.

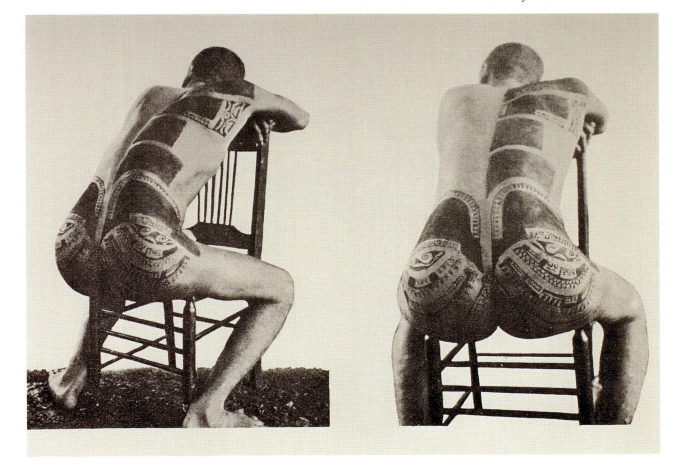

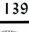

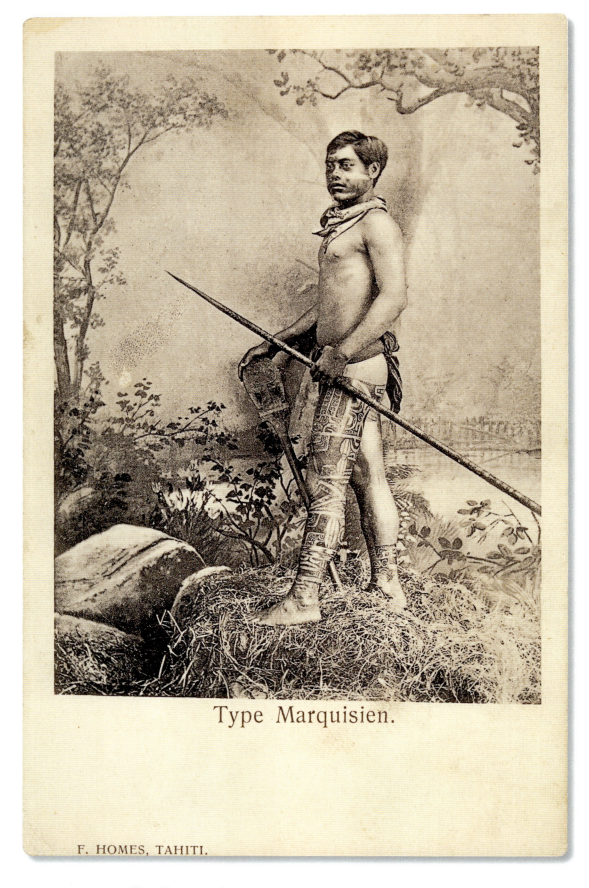

Type Marquisien.

F. HOMES, TAHITI.

"Type Marquisien." A studio portrait that was one of the most popular images available at the time depicting traditional tattooing of the Marquesas. In this image the leg tattoos are of the classic style, which is quite unusual considering the late date and the fact that the male depicted appears to be quite young. Original postcard published by Frank Homes circa 1905.

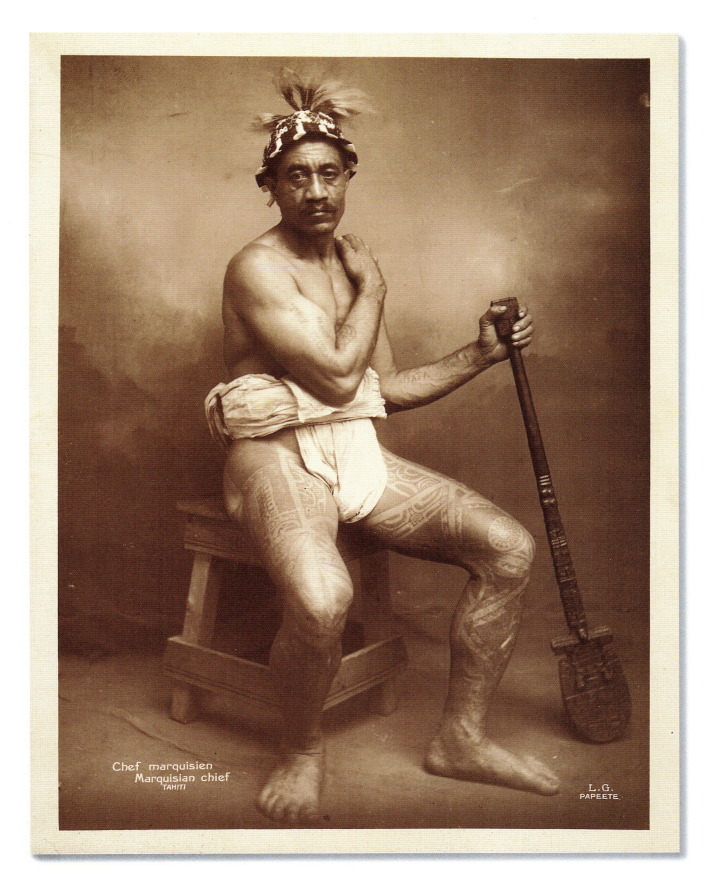

Original photograph entitled "Marquesan Chief-Tahiti." From a series of sepia photographs by Lucien Gauthier* circa 1919. In this "staged" studio portrait, along with the traditional Marquesan tattooing the man is wearing several unusual arm tattoos with wording similar to Maori memorial and baptismal tattoos. On his head is an ornament made of clam and turtle shell carved with *tiki* figures in motif. The head ornament called *Paekaha* is adorned at the top with strands of gray hair from old men's beards. The *U'u* club he is resting his hand on is a late example made for the curio market.

*Lucien Gauthier (1875-1971) was a important photographer and artist, arriving from France in 1904 and setting up a commercial photo studio in Papeete Tahiti at the hotel Tiare. Best known for his photographic postcards and studio portraits he became like Spitz and Homes, a dealer in all sorts of island curios. He was also known for his work and association with the artist Matisse during his brief visit to Tahiti and French Polynesia in 1930.

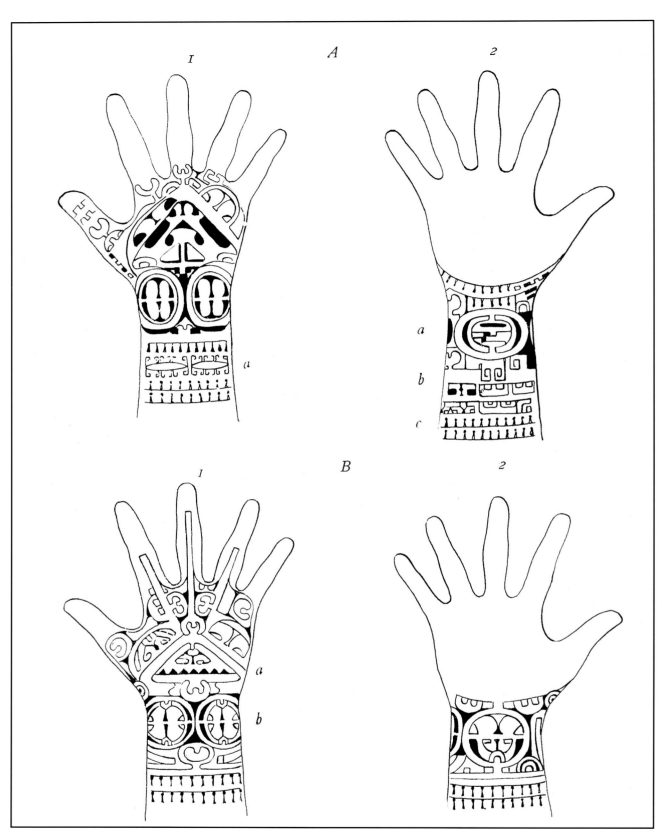

Drawing entitled "Tattoo Designs in the Marquesas." From Willowdean Chatterson Handy's classic account published by Bishop Museum in 1921 entitled *Tattooing in the Marquesas*. In this illustration hand patterns from Tahu Ata and Hiva Oa are shown. Plate A shows a hand of a woman of Fatu Hiva: #1 The back of the hand, #2 the palm, showing the *pariho* motif on the underwrist around the area of the palm, the *mata* (a), the *tamau* (b) and the *pariho* (c). Plate B shows a hand of a woman from Tahu Ata: #1 The back, showing the *poka'a* motif at the base of the middle finger, the *pihau* (a) and the *mata* (b), #2 the underwrist.

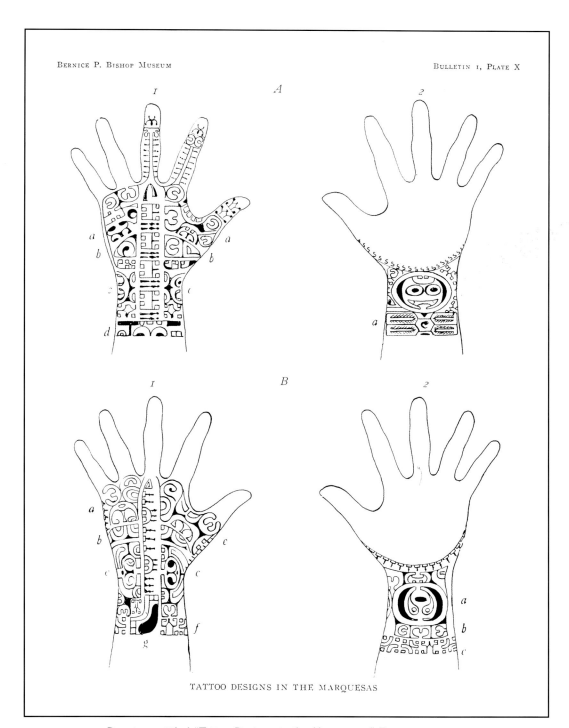

Drawing entitled "Tattoo Designs in the Marquesas." From Willowdean Chatterson Handy's classic account published by Bishop Museum in 1921 entitled *Tattooing in the Marquesas*. In this illustration hand patterns from the island of Tahu Ata are shown: Plate A depicts the back of the hand showing the *ka'ava* motif at the base of the middle finger to the wrist, *kou'u* (a) *poka'a* (b) *mohovaha* (c) and the *mata* (d), #2 the underwrist with the *koua'ehi* motif (a). Plate B depicts the back of the hand showing the following patterns *papua* (a) *e tua poou* (b) *paka* (c) *ka'ava* (center) *fanaua* (e) *Pohu* (f) and *ka'ake* (g). #2 on the underwrist shows the pattern *paa niho* around the palm: *papua au ti* (b) and the *vai o Kena*.

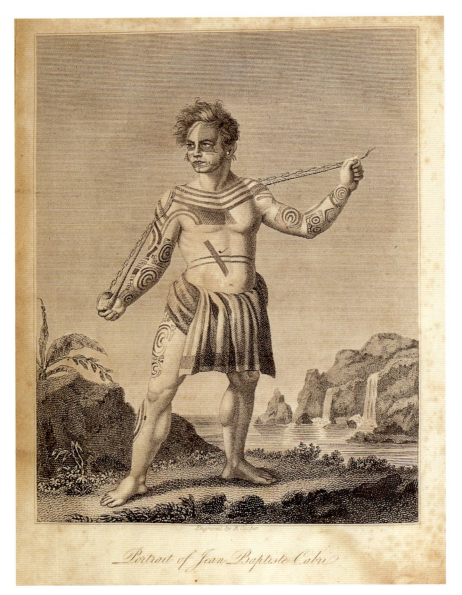

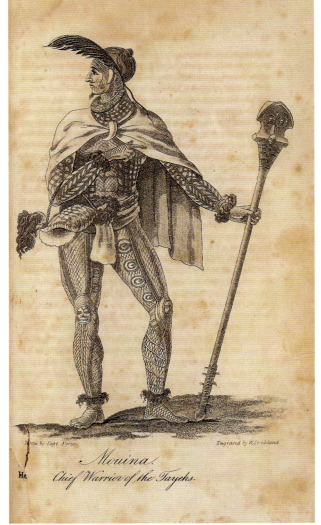

Engraving entitled "Portrait of Jean Baptiste Cabri." From G.H. Von Langsdorff's Russian voyage of exploration published in 1813 in London. This wonderful and rather amusing illustration depicts the Frenchman Jean Baptiste Cabri who was the first recorded European to be tattooed in the Marquesas, having obtained the tattoos after jumping ship. Cabri was well known for creating problems between European traders and explorers who passed through the islands. After leaving the Marquesas some years later he made a living travelling throughout Europe and Russia displaying his tattoos and entertaining groups with his South Sea tales. After his death in Brittany in 1822 his skin was preserved and displayed - a rather gruesome legacy. In this image Cabri's eyes are decorated with striated lines that were identified as *mata toetoe* motif and said to identify members of the *Ka'ioi** - whether this is true remains to be seen.

*The *Ka'ioi* were dancing troupes composed of both males and females and were an important part of Marquesan society.

Engraving entitled "Mouina – Chief Warrior of the Tayehs." From Captain David Porter's *Journal of a Cruise made to the Pacific Ocean in the United States Frigate "Essex" in the years 1812-1814* and published in two volumes in Philadelphia in 1822. This illustration shows the chief warrior in full tattoo with all his regalia – Captain Porter describes him as follows: "He was a tall, well shaped man of about thirty-five years of age, remarkably active, of an intelligent and open countenance, and his whole appearance was prepossessing."

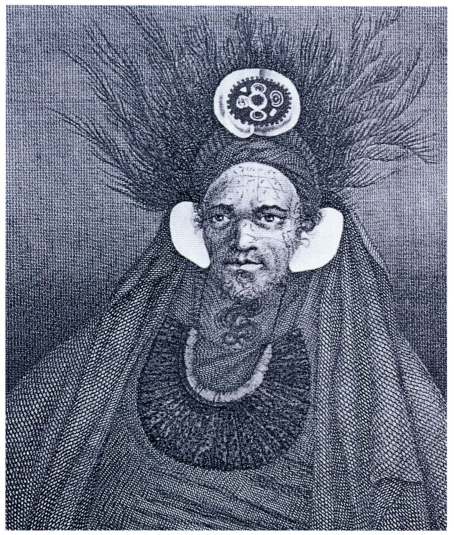

Engraving entitled "The Chief at St. Christina."* Published in the atlas to Cook's second voyage, this drawing is attributed to William Hodges and is the first known illustration of tattoo on a Marquesan Islander.
*St. Christina was the 18th century name for the island of Tahuata in the Marquesan group.

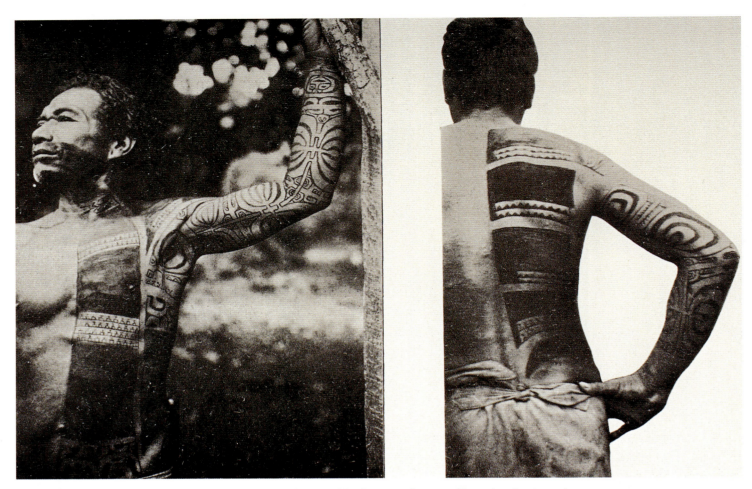

Photographs showing front and back views of a man. From the classic work on the Marquesas by Karl von den Steinen *Die Marquesaner und ihre Kunst*, published in Germany in 1925. These photos of a man from Hiva Oa shows upper body tattoos including what appears to be a facial tattoo by the Marquesan name of *ti' i – nutu* as labeled by Von Den Steinen.

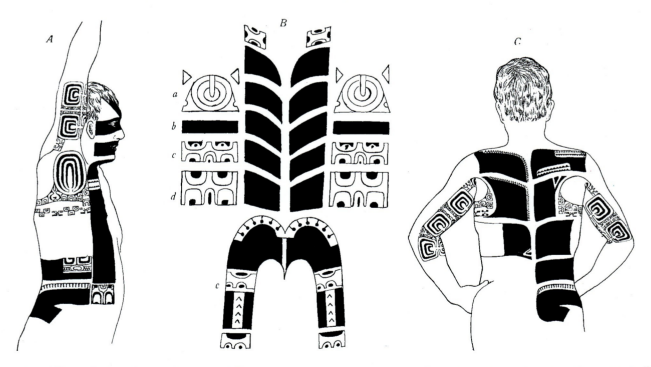

Drawing entitled "Tattoo Designs in the Marquesas." From Willowdean Chatterson Handy's classic account published by Bishop Museum in 1921 entitled *Tattooing in the Marquesas*. In this illustration body patterns for men are depicted in what Handy calls "old and new types." Plate A shows an unfinished example that she says was typical of all the islands at the time she recorded it and depicts the armpit design *ipu katu* and chest *teeva*. Plate B shows what Handy labels as "very old patterns" from the island of Fatu Hiva and were made after a drawing from a *Tuhuna* of that island showing back patterns *pahito; ipu oto* (a) *pahito* (b) *mata* (c) *mata* (d) *kohe tua* (e) a girdle and leg stripe. Plate C illustrates an unfinished back pattern *peka tua* from Nuku Hiva, but common to all islands according to Handy. On Ua Pou she records that the same pattern as *moho*.

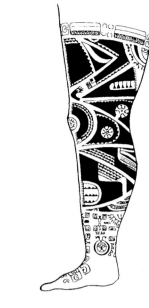
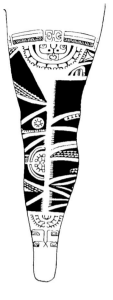

Drawing entitled "Tattoo Designs in the Marquesas." From Willowdean Chatterson Handy's classic account published by Bishop Museum in 1921 entitled *Tattooing in the Marquesas*. In this illustration leg patterns are shown that Handy described as the only known surviving example of their type and of an "old style." These were recorded on the island of Nuku Hiva.

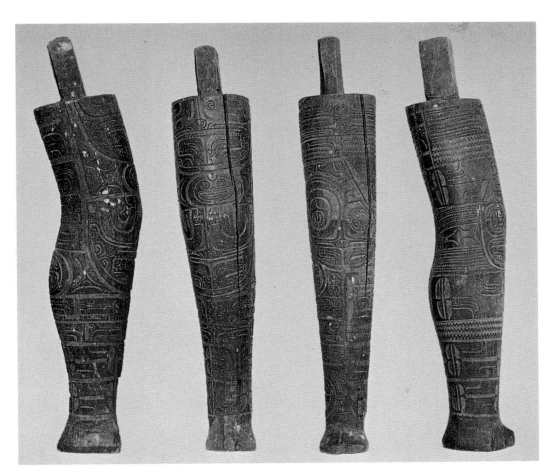

Original photograph labeled "Tattoo wood model legs." The carvings depicted here have always been described in literature as a type of model or pattern for the artist to follow. Although remotely possible, the author believes more than likely they were simply a curio made at the end of the last century for sale to the occasional visitor.

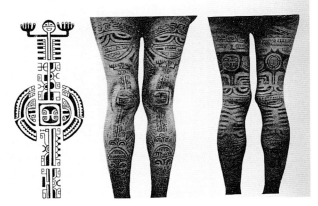

Photograph of a woman's legs, front and back. From the classic work on the Marquesas by Karl von den Steinen *Die Marquesaner und ihre Kunst*, published in Germany in 1925. Observed on a woman on the island of Ua Pou in the village of Hakahau, also illustrated is an artist rendering of the front legs with unusual *tiki* motif.

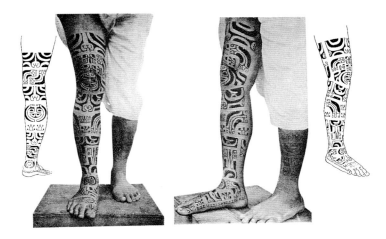

Photograph of a woman's legs, front and side view. From the classic work on the Marquesas by Karl von den Steinen *Die Marquesaner und ihre Kunst*, published in Germany in 1925. This woman was quite famous for her tattooed legs, having been photographed by the female photographer Mrs. S. Hoare in Papeete Tahiti in 1892. She was also sketched and painted by several artists as early as 1888. Known as "Frau Bradora," her legs are shown here in great detail. Von den Steinen recorded the tattoo motif on her knee as *kautupa,* an abstract face-like motif.

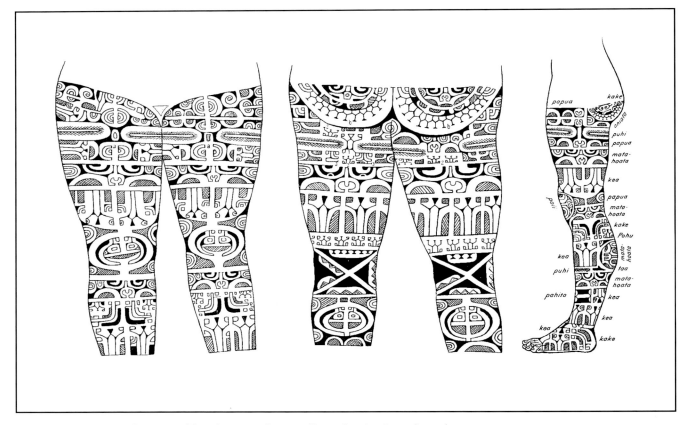

Drawing of female tattoo designs. From the classic work on the Marquesas by Karl von den Steinen *Die Marquesaner und ihre Kunst*, published in Germany in 1925. A detailed drawing with their accompanying Marquesan names showing design elements of the legs and thighs on a woman of Hiva Oa.

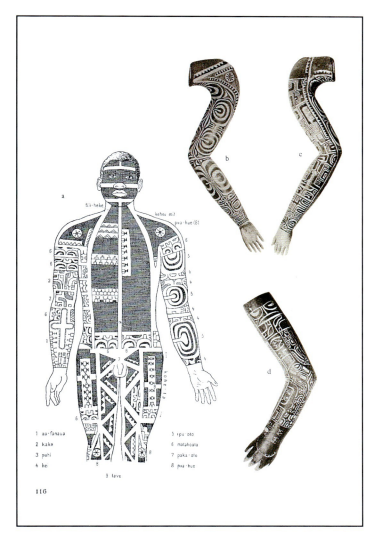

Drawing of male tattoo designs. From the classic work on the Marquesas by Karl von den Steinen *Die Marquesaner und ihre Kunst*, published in Germany in 1925. A detailed drawing with accompanying Marquesan names showing design elements on a man of Hiva Oa.

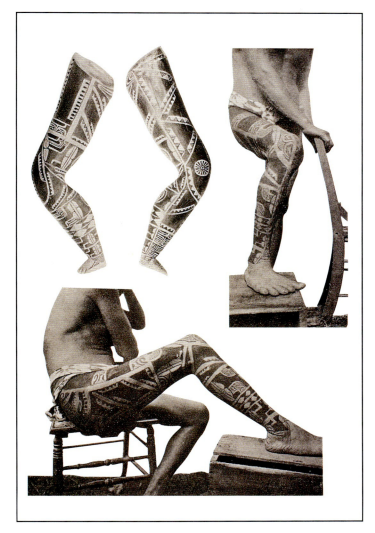

Photograph of a man's leg, front and side views. From the classic work on the Marquesas by Karl von den Steinen *Die Marquesaner und ihre Kunst*, published in Germany in 1925. This series of photographs shows two views of a leg of a man from Nuku Hiva.

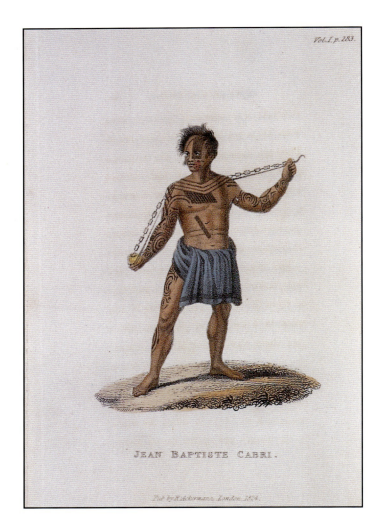

Left: Engraving entitled "Jean Baptiste Cabri." Another colored version from *The World in Miniature – South Sea Islands*, published in 1824 in London, Frederick Shorbel editor.

Below: Drawings entitled "Tattoo designs in the Marquesas." From Willowdean Chatterson Handy's classic account published by Bishop Museum in 1921 entitled *Tattooing in the Marquesas*. In this drawing face patterns for men are shown. #1 shows an unfinished example from Hiva Oa, #2 shows *enata* motif from the island of Ua Pou, #3 shows a half band on forehead from Ua Pou, #4 shows the following motifs *tiki ae* (a) *kikomata* (b) *tiki pu* (c) and *pariho* (inset in c) all recorded on the island of Ua Huka, #5 shows a band over one eye *mata* and mouth band *nutu kaha* recorded on Hiva Oa, #6 shows the following designs elements *vahana ae* (a) *mata* (b) *nihoniho peata* (c left) name unknown (c right) *kikutu* (d and e) all recorded on Ua Huka, #7 and #8 are also from Ua Huka.

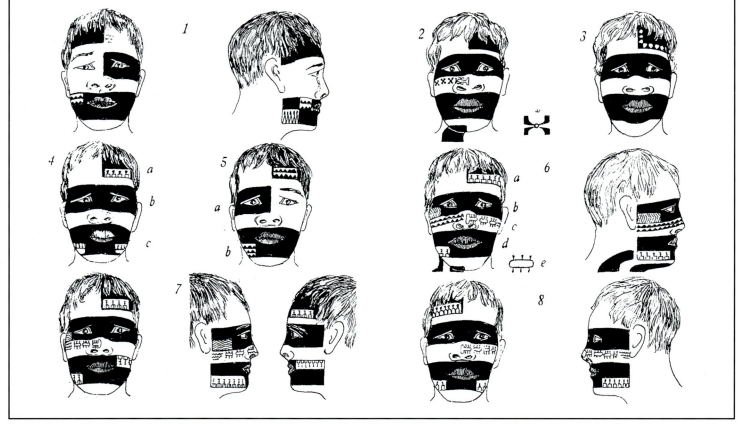

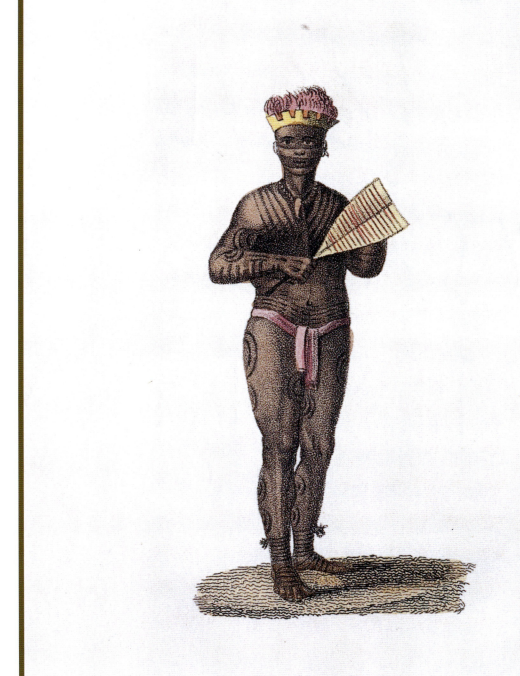

Engraving entitled "Native of La Magdelena – *(Marquesas Islands)* with a Fan." From *The World in Miniature – South Sea Islands*, published in 1824 in London, Frederick Shorbel editor. A rare print showing a type of tattoo not usually seen in depictions of this time period.

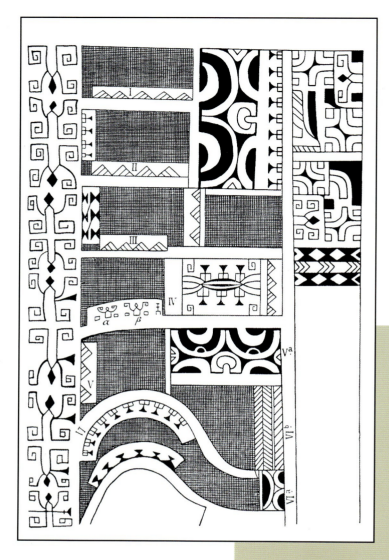

Drawing of male tattoo designs. From the classic work on the Marquesas by Karl von den Steinen *Die Marquesaner und ihre Kunst*, published in Germany in 1925. This series of very detailed drawings shows, in the upper illustration neck and throat designs and, to the right, the back of an upper arm design. The lower drawing shows, to the left, buttock and thigh designs, while the right shows buttock and upper arm designs. These tattoo motifs were seen on the island of Hiva Oa.

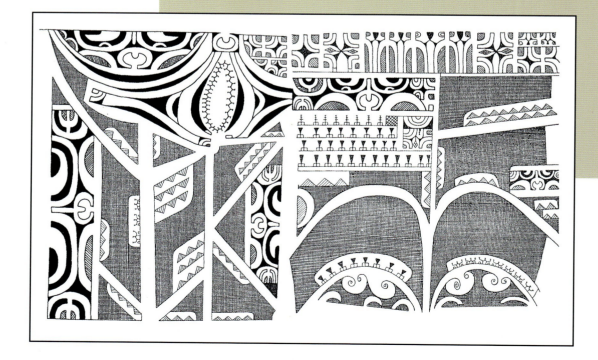

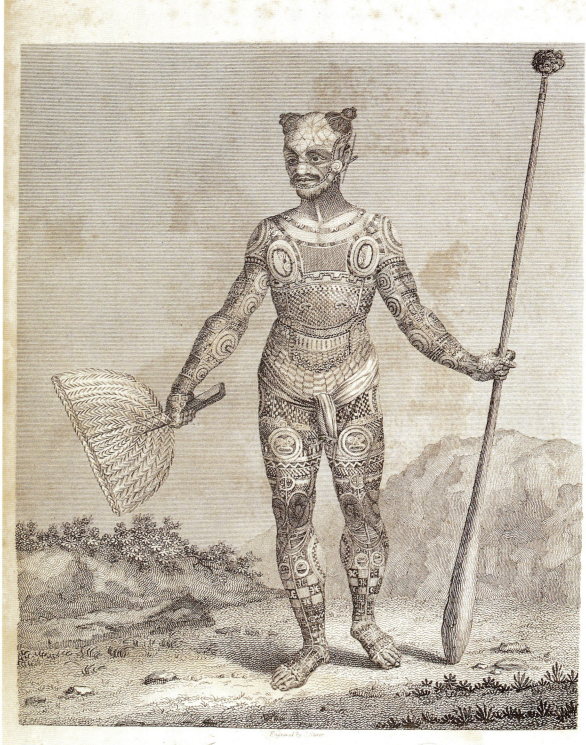

Engraving entitled "An inhabitant of the island of Nukahiva." From G. H. Von Langsdorff's Russian voyage of exploration published in 1813 in London. Drawn from life, it is very accurate in the placement of tattoo motifs and designs although as always a bit of artistic license is used. In his right hand he is holding a ceremonial staff *Toko toko pio'o,* the top bundle of the staff with curled human hair pompon terminal. In his other hand is a fan, an item indicating prestige and chiefly rank.

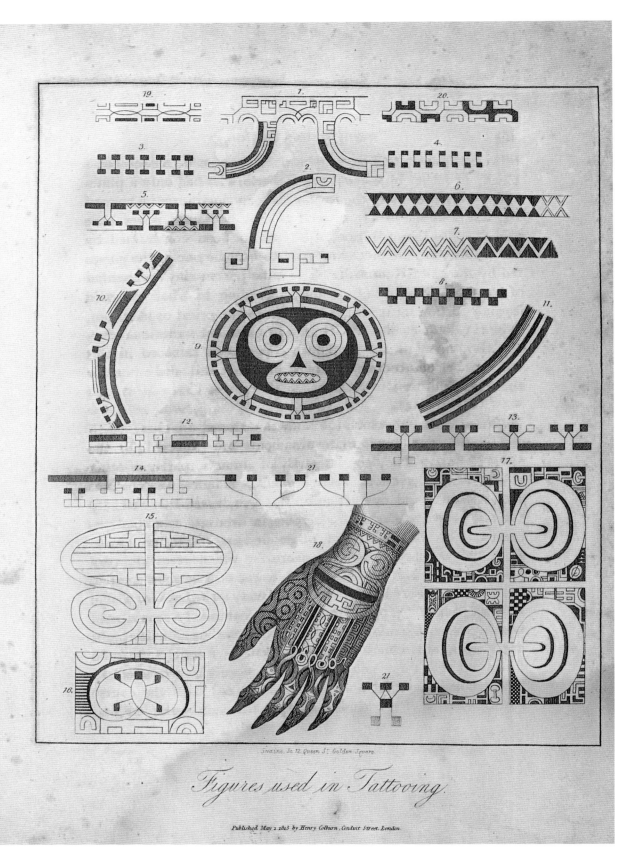

Engraving entitled "Figures used in Tattooing." From G.H. Von Langsdorff's Russian voyage of exploration published in 1813 in London. This is one of the earliest published accounts of traditional Marquesan tattooing, showing design elements in great detail.

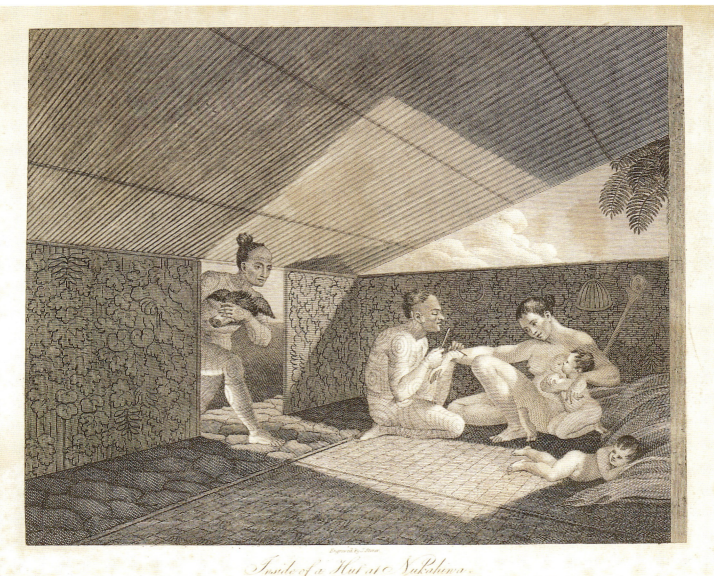

Engraving entitled "Inside of a Hut at Nukahiva." From G.H. Von Langsdorff's Russian voyage of exploration published in 1813 in London. This is the earliest known image of the actual process of tattooing in Polynesia. Here is shown a rather fanciful illustration depicting the tattoo artist at work with his tools. It is interesting to note the person entering the hut is carrying a pig in his arm presumably in payment for the tattoo artist's work.

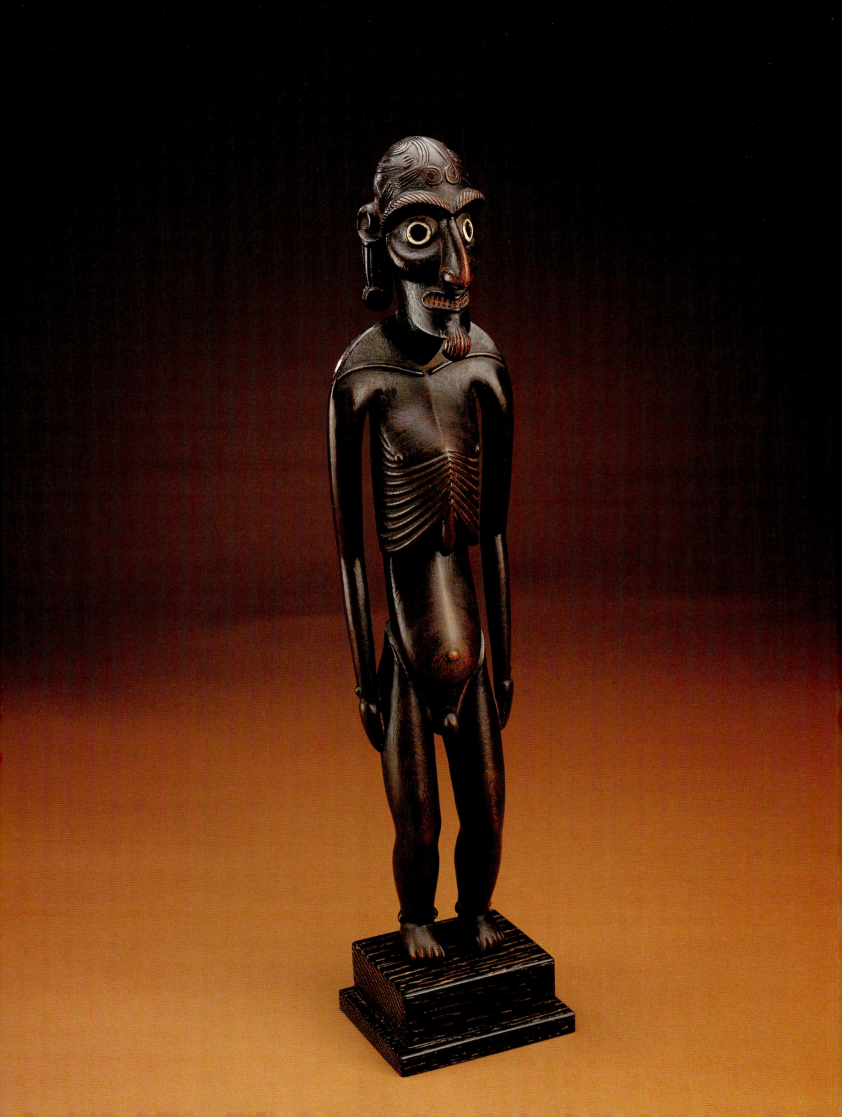

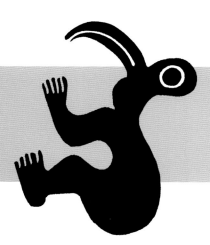

EASTER ISLAND
Rapa Nui

Of all the islands in Polynesia there is probably no island or group of islands as mysterious as Easter Island. Lying over 2,000 miles from the South American coast and 1,700 miles from Mangareva, it is the most isolated and forsaken of all the islands in Polynesia. The island is volcanic in origin and composed primarily of soft volcanic rock. Several smooth-sided extinct cones rise in various places on the island with outcroppings of basalt and obsidian providing a varied resource of workable stone. Total land area on the island is approximately 50 square miles making it an area of very limited resources. Rainfall averages around 55 inches per year but is quickly absorbed in the porous soil, leaving the primary sources of water the crater lakes found on Rano Kau. One of the coolest climates in Polynesia, the temperature varies from approximately 60 to 72 degrees Fahrenheit with the weather being very unsettled in the winter months. Vegetation on the island is sparse, with trees of any size being a rarity;[1] the island today is covered by a coarse grass being suitable for one of the principal occupations on the island in this century – sheep ranching. The first Polynesian settlers introduced crop plants such as taro, sugarcane and bananas – along with the main staple, the sweet potato.[2] Domesticated fowls, an important source of food, were also brought by the first settlers - along with several unintentional stowaways: the lizard and the rat.

The first settlers originated in the Marquesas,[3] arriving sometime after 400 AD with additional settlements being unlikely due to the island's remote location.[4] According to Rapanui[5] traditions, the chief of this first voyaging canoe was Hotu Matua, leading his tribe ashore at Anakena. After a long period of isolation this population steadily began increasing, resulting in various family lineage groups being formed. These groups or *kainga* claimed their own territorial areas, all being ritually

Left: Male figure *moai kava kava*. Carved of toromiro wood with bird bone and obsidian eyes, this remarkable sculpture is one of the most extraordinary creations in Polynesia. Beautifully carved with fine detailing, these more than likely represent ancestor figures who reappeared to the living as ghosts.* According to reports gathered during the 19th century, these figures were occasionally suspended around the neck by high-ranking males during important egg gathering and fishing events, with a single individual having as many as twenty carvings adorning his person and, in the process, gathering status from both the number in his possession and the quality of their carving. The present figure is one of the finest of its kind. The superb sculptural detailing of the face, with its jutting chin, high cheekbones, protruding nose, as well as the fine carving of the skeletal components, provide it with a supernatural presence. 18th century. Height 18-3/4 inches. Traces of red pigment on surface. Formerly in the collections of Pike; Sotheby's - New York; Merton Simpson, New York; Hemmeter, Honolulu; Bonhams, London; Private collection, Barcelona Spain.

*There has always been a great deal of debate among scholars as to the actual use and meaning of these figures. Francina Forment has recently postulated that the beak-like treatment of the nose and the recurrent imagery of the frigate bird on top of the heads of many examples, including this one, may symbolize the birdman deity. The use of bird bone inlays in the eyes and the disk shape in the back of the pelvis, which she compares to the vulvae of birds, provide further connections to a human avian being.

Right: Drawing of a frigate bird motif. The glyph illustrated here is carved in relief on the top of the *moai kava kava's* head. This design was seen in various forms and was tattooed on both sexes symbolizing the birdman deity, an important figure in Rapanui mythology.

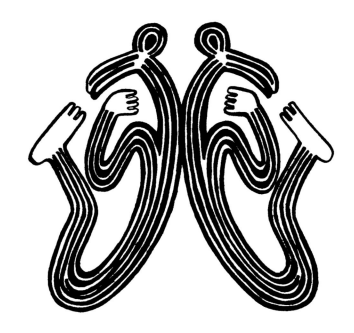

by construction of temples or *ahu*. Although sharing features similar to those of Hawai`i and Tahiti in construction, the Rapanui incorporated the carving of stone images representing deified ancestors. These statues or *moai*[6] were erected upon the stone foundations of these temples with sizes increasing over time due to the improved technical skills of the carvers and a competition among the various lineages to see who could erect the largest statues. A marked growth in the population resulted in a shortage of natural resources causing further problems among the various groups leading to frequent warfare[7] and a state of general turmoil and confusion.

People of senior rank known as *ariki* were subject to customary restrictions and regulations with a set of complex *mana* and *tapu* regulations governing the behavior of the general populace. Priests or *ivi atua* acted as intermediaries between humans and gods, with the god Makemake being the most prominent.[8] This god was associated with the birdman cult and involved elaborate rituals and offerings, the most important being the festival held at Orongo. In this festival competitors gathered and sent a representative or *hopu* to swim to nearby Motu Nui islet to search for the first egg of the season laid by the sooty tern. The first person finding an egg and bringing it back undamaged was the "birdman" for the year and was vested with considerable power and prestige during this period.[9]

Houses best described as being in the shape of an overturned boat with an upward pointing keel were constructed on stone foundations with wood framework and reed or grass thatching. Like elsewhere in Polynesia, specialists, craftsman or *maori* were employed in a variety of fields. Women were involved in a variety of pursuits including the production of barkcloth known as *tapa*, the paper mulberry plant[10] being cultivated in special stone enclosures. A *tapa* cloak was worn by both sexes with an additional wraparound skirt worn by the women, and everyday clothing consisting of a small loincloth of grass. Feather headdresses were occasionally worn by men, with various ear ornaments and necklaces worn by both sexes.

With no sheltered harbors along its coasts, Easter Island provides no safe anchorage,[11] yet in 1722 on Easter Day, April 5, the Dutch explorer Jacob Roggeveen (1659-1729)[12] anchored along the north coast of the island, probably at La Perouse. The following is an excerpt from his journal and gives us a good description of the first encounter with the Rapanui:

> They had seen very distinctly ahead to starboard a low flat island… We gave to… The land of the name of the Paasch Eyland (Easter Island), because it was discovered and found by us on Easter Day… In the morning Captain Bouman… Brought to our ship a Paaschlander with his vessel who was quite naked, without having the least covering in front of what modesty forbids being named more clearly. This poor person appeared to be very glad to see us, and marvelled greatly at the construction of our ship… After we had amused ourselves enough with him, and he with us, we sent him back to shore in his canoe, having been presented with two blue strings of beads round his neck, a small mirror, a pair of scissors, and other such trifles, in which he seemed to take special pleasure and satisfaction…Very many canoes came to the ships. These people showed at this time their great eagerness for all they saw and were so bold that they took the hats and caps of the sailors from their heads and jumped overboard,[13] for they are extremely good swimmers, as was shown by the fact that a large number came swimming from land to the ships… We set out in the morning with three boats and two sloops, manned with 134 men, and all armed with a musket, cartridge pouch and sword… we marched forward a little… to our great astonishment and without any expectation it was heard that four to five musket-shots from behind us were made… more than thirty muskets were let off, and the Indians being completely surprised and frightened by this fled, leaving behind 10 to 12 dead, besides the wounded… The Under Mate… came to me saying that… one of the inhabitants grasped the muzzle of his musket in order to take it from him by force, whom he pushed back; then that another Indian tried to pull the coat of a sailor off his body, and that some of the inhabitants, seeing our resistance, picked up some stones with a menacing gesture of throwing at us, by which by all appearance the shooting by my small troop had been caused… After a lapse of a little time they brought a large quantity of sugarcane, fowls, yams, and bananas; but we gave them to understand by signs that we wanted nothing except only the fowls, being about 60 in number, and 30 bunches of bananas, for which we paid them the value amply with striped linen, with which they appeared to be well pleased and satisfied… The ears of these people from youth are… stretched in the lobes and the innermost part cut out… Now when these Indians have to do something, and these ear pendants through swinging hither and thither would be troublesome to them, they take them off and pull the opening of the lobe up over the edge of the ear, which makes a strange laughable appearnce… These people have snow-white teeth, and are outstandingly strong in the teeth… Concerning the religon of these people, of this we could get no full knowledge because of the shortness of our stay; we merely observed that they set fires before some particularly high erected stone images, and then sitting down on their heels with bowed heads, they bring the palms of their hands together, bringing them up and down. These stone images at first caused us to be struck with astonishment, because we could not comprehend how it was possible that these people, who are devoid of thick timber for making any machines, as well as strong ropes, nevertheless had been able to erect such images, which were fully 30 feet high and thick in proportion.[14]

The exchanges became friendly for the rest of their stay with no further exploration of the island attempted. Roggeveen, fearing for the safety of his vessels when a northerly wind blew up, decided to leave the island and sailed forth on the tenth of April, ending a sad chapter in the island's history.

The next brief visit was by the Spanish under Felipe Gonzalez (1703-1792) with his two ships stopping for six days in 1770 and taking possession of the Island for Spain. It was the celebrated navigator Captain James Cook who visited the island during his second voyage in 1774 who led the first survey of the island, a party of men venturing inland making observations. The Frenchman La Perouse traced these steps arriving in 1786. In 1804 the first of several raids on the local populace began with the American schooner *Nancy* kidnapping twenty-two islanders for a seal hunting expedition to the Juan Fernandez Islands. This tragedy ended when, after three days sailing, the prisoners were allowed on deck - only to jump overboard swimming in the direction of their island home. Despite numerous attempts to try and save them, they all perished at sea. This event did not stop the Captain from organizing additional raids on the island and recruiting men by force. This crime, known as "Blackbirding," continued periodically throughout the first half of the 19th century making the islanders very distrustful and hostile to any new visitors - mostly whalers and traders. In 1862 a final and devastating blow was dealt to the people and culture of the island when Peruvian ships recruiting labor for the guano islands kidnapped over two hundred islanders including many leaders and learned people.[15] The few surviving islanders that were able to return from this forced slavery brought with them smallpox and influenza, further decimating the entire population.[16] By 1877 the population had been tragically reduced with only 111 Rapanui surviving from an estimated 9500 at the time of contact.

The Catholic Church established a mission upon the island in 1863/64 resulting in more frequent visits from foreigners. Chile annexed the island in 1888 and in 1901 the entire area except for the village of Hanga Roa was turned over to the Chilean Navy with the majority of the land leased to the firm of Williamson and Balfour for sheep ranching. This large operation continued for many years until it was taken over by the Navy - with the last of the sheep being sold off in the early 1980s.[17] Finally in 1966, a Chilean decree created a new province: Easter Island, province of Valparaiso. Today the island is under a new threat with a burgeoning population of over 2500 people, making the current economic climate bleak – the only real source of income being tourism. Easter Island's rich cultural heritage and sites are the economic answer for the islanders but the challenge of exploding growth in this area must be met with a sound ecological approach and plan; if not, the great mysteries of the island may be lost forever.

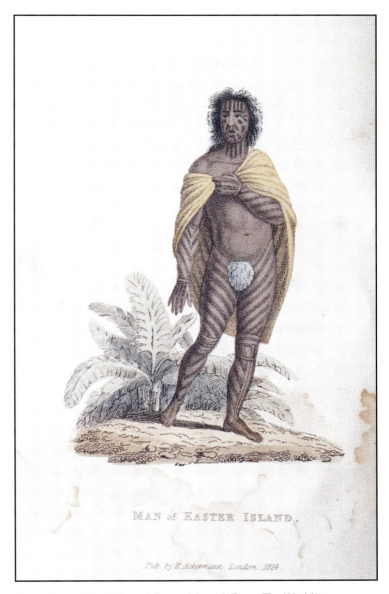

Engraving entitled "Man of Easter Island." From *The World in Miniature – South Sea Islands*, published in 1824 in London, Frederick Shorbel editor. A unique depiction of tattooing on Easter Island with a tremendous amount of artistic license.

Easter Island Chronology*

Early Period – 400-1100 AD
The initial phase of settling and development, with statues erected before 700. These statues are small and, according to Van Tilburg, of two or possibly three morphological types. At the end of this phase there is an *ahu* on the site of Orongo.

Middle Period – 1100-1680
This period is known as an age of expansion or *Ahu Moai* phase, with the architecture reaching its peak at the start of this period. The *ahu* grow in size; the *moai* erected upon these *ahu* platforms become more stereotyped, growing larger and larger in size. The size increases, probably as a result of increased competition between the lineages, marking the preeminence of chiefs over priests. Based upon archaeological evidence, it is estimated that the population in the year 1600 is 9,000. At Orongo around the year 1400, stone houses are built, oval in shape, but the oldest dwellings with thick drystone walls date after 1540.

Late Period – 1680-1722
Known as the decadent period or *Huri Moai* phase, this represents a time when no *ahu moai* are constructed, with most of them having been destroyed or abandoned. Semi-pyramidal *ahu* are built and used as tombs. The opposition between the east and west territorial entities becomes flagrant, while the birdman cult develops. This phase ended with Roggeveen's arrival in 1722.

Protohistoric Period – 1722-1868
The *ahu* continue to be used as tombs; contact with Europeans brings massive changes. The population is estimated at around 9,000 at the time of contact, and 8,200 in the year 1850. The end of this phase coincides with the conversion to Christianity.

Historic Period - 1868-Present
At the start of this period, the population is concentrated at the southwest part of the island. By 1877 there are only 111 remaining islanders left following the abductions by Peruvian slavers, the epidemics and the departure of the islanders for Tahiti. The *ahu*, sometimes used as tombs at the beginning of the 20th century, lose their religious functions completely. Annexation by Chili in 1888 and the beginning of excessive tourism in the 1990s.

*This chronology based upon dating by Michel Orliac, Paris.

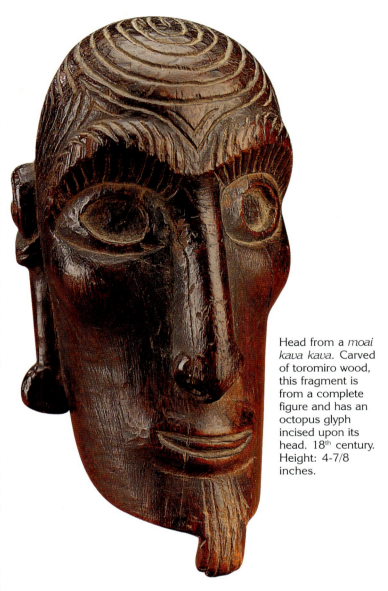

Head from a *moai kava kava*. Carved of toromiro wood, this fragment is from a complete figure and has an octopus glyph incised upon its head. 18th century. Height: 4-7/8 inches.

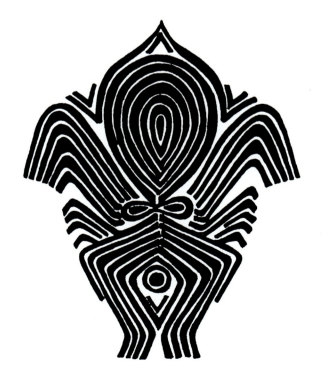

Drawing of an octopus motif. The glyph illustrated here is incised on the top of the head the fragmentary *moai kava kava*. This design was used in tattoo patterns and is also found in rock art of the island.

Easter Island Tattooing – *ta'*

Oral traditions provide a mythological origin for the art of tattoo on Easter Island, with the two female spirits *Vi'e Moko* and *Vi'e Kena* and their sons providing the basis for the myth. The actual origin for the custom may lie in the simple fact that the art was brought with the first settlers from the Marquesas and adapted into their own unique Rapanui style.[18] Which of these, if any, is the actual source for the tradition may never be known, thus remaining another mystery of the island.

The process of tattooing on Easter Island was similar to other areas in Polynesia. Pigment was made from burnt ti leaves[19] and incorporated similar tools, such as the adze-like bone comb known as *uhi* and the wood mallet. It was Captain Cook who visited the island on his second voyage in 1774 that has left us with one of the best accounts of a Rapanui:

> I did not see a Man in this Isle that measured Six feet, in generall they are a very slender race but very Nimble and Active, well featured with agreeable countenances, but as much addicted to theiving as their Neighbours; Tattowing that is inlaying the Colour of black in the Skin is much used here, the Men are coloured in this manner from head to foot, the figures they mark are all nearly alike only some give them one direction on the boddy and some nother according to fancy, they also make use of Red and White Paint, to their faces and sometimes to other parts of their bodies, the former is made of Tamrick but what the latter is made of I know not.

Women were also seen with tattoos on the same voyage as reported by Forster:

> They are all prodigously tattooed on every part of the body, the face in particular; and all their women... had likewise punctures on the face, which resembled patches worn by our ladies.

Tattoo motifs used were varied according to one's position held in society or were of a more personal nature. Like the Marquesas, tattooing was a lengthy process, taking place at different periods in one's life, the first tattoos being applied with the onset of puberty. Patterns were primarily linear in design with triangular and circular elements occasionally interspersed. Realistic motifs were also an important part of the repertoire often marking important events in one's own life, as was reported by Metraux,[20] who records a woman with a *rapa*[21] tattooed on her back representing her first lover. Other observers also recorded designs marking events in one's life, such as the *komari*[22] design seen by Geiseler[23] distinguishing a married man. Many designs were inspired by myths[24] such as the birdman. A wide range of other more realistic motifs were also used including obsidian spear heads, plants, *moai*, fishhooks, houses, boats, human figures and chickens.

The art of tattoo was shortly abandoned after the arrival of the first missionaries in 1863/64 and was virtually non-existent by the time the American ship *Mohican* arrived in 1886. Spending fourteen days on the island, paymaster William Thomson[25] left us with the following account:

> Tattooing is not practised at the present time, none being observed upon children and young persons. But all those advanced in life are ornamented on all parts of the body. Unlike the Samoans and other islanders, where a standard pattern is adhered to, the designs were only limited by the fancy and ability of the artist.

Tattooing on Easter Island has been making a revival in the last two decades, incorporating traditional motifs as well as new patterns inspired by items outside the traditional culture, all now being permanently marked in tattooers' ink on the skin of many modern-day Rapanui.

Endnotes

[1] A species of mimosa (*Sophora toromiro*) grew on the island at the time of contact, providing a source of wood used in traditional carving. Recent archaeological findings on the island also indicate the existence of large areas of coconut palms.

[2] The sweet potato (*kumara; Ipomoea batatas*) has been a point of contention in the debate among the academic community as to when the first inhabitants arrived and where they originated.

[3] There is a remote possibility that the southern Cook Islands or Austral Islands were the point of origin.

[4] Thor Heyerdahl, noted explorer and author, has suggested that the original settlers of Easter Island originated in South America. He is most famous for his *Kon Tiki* voyage attempting to show contact was possible between the two distant cultures. The voyage proved that it is possible to traverse vast distances in such flimsy craft, but the actual likelihood of arriving in Easter Island is at best very remote due to wind and current conditions, which favor an arrival in the Marquesas or Tuamotu group. The author, though disagreeing with his arguments for a South American connection, still has a great deal of admiration and respect for this truly remarkable man.

[5] Rapa Nui or Big Rapa is the name given to the island in historic times when some Polynesians working as sailors on whaling ships came to the island. It reminded them of Rapa Iti (Little Rapa), a smaller island 700 miles south-southwest. The general consensus is that the people of Easter Island never had a name for their island; it was "the land," as it was the only island they knew. All the names now known for the island were given by outsiders, including "Naval of the World." When there is a group of islands and interchange between them, one needs an identifier or name. When there is only one island and no contact with the outside world, the naming of the island is not important. Personal communication, Dr. Georgia Lee.

[6] These monolithic sculptures are Easter Island's most recognizable landmarks and have been subjected to a great deal of attention among scholars and the general public.

[7] A class of professional warriors known as the *matatoa* was maintained for war, with disputes often being centered on minor *tapu* violations and personal insults.

[8] The other gods in the pantheon of the Rapanui were Tane, Rongo, Tu and Tangaroa. These gods or *atua* appeared as only legendary figures unlike other areas in Polynesia.

[9] Many birdman petroglyphs exist on the island especially at Orongo. Tattoo motifs also appear to relate to this ritual with Metraux recording several patterns.

[10] The paper mulberry *Broussonetia papyrifera* was one of the plants imported to the island by the first Polynesian settlers.

[11] Having no sheltered harbors, unpredictable winds and ocean currents combined with the island's isolation, lack of resources and suspicious attitude of the Rapanui people, the island proved to be too dangerous for ships and men, resulting in infrequent contact in the 18th and early 19th centuries.

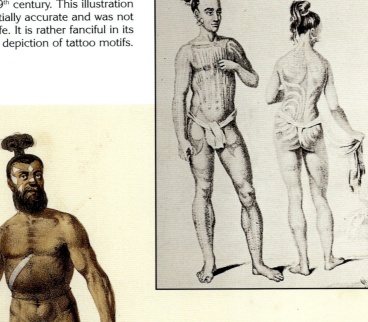

Engraving of Easter Islanders. Drawn by the artist Rienzi in the 19th century. This illustration is probably only partially accurate and was not drawn from life. It is rather fanciful in its depiction of tattoo motifs.

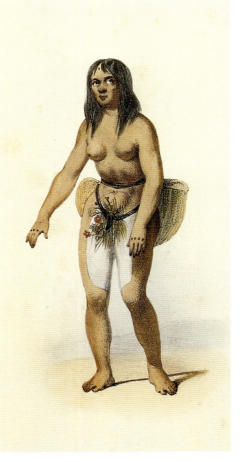

Engraving of Easter Islanders. Drawn from life by the artist Louis Choris on Kotzebue's voyage around the world in the years 1815-1818. This beautiful engraving shows a fairly accurate depiction of traditional male tattoo as it appeared during the first half of the 19th century. Published as part of a separate atlas in 1822.

[12] Roggeveen's exploration of the Pacific from east to west proved to be one of the more unfortunate and tragic voyages in the annals of Pacific exploration. His fleet of ships encountered shipwrecks, desertion and scurvy, with the latter killing more than fifty percent of his crew.
[13] This was a common occurrence throughout the islands of Polynesia at the time of contact, with the Polynesian concept of private ownership being virtually non-existent.
[14] *The Journal of Jacob Roggeveen*, translated and edited by Andrew Sharp in 1970.
[15] In this unscrupulous and deceitful act all the expert knowledge of the traditional culture died with the unfortunate victims on the Peruvian coastal islands, resulting in the present-day lack of knowledge on many aspects of traditional Rapanui culture.
[16] In 1870 a further blow to the population occurred when a large number of the islanders left to work in the plantations of Tahiti.
[17] Cattle and horses have replaced the sheep, creating many problems - currently there is not enough feed and water on the island to support the livestock.
[18] Geiseler reported in the 1880s that tattooing was unknown prior to the time of contact, being brought to the island by a Marquesan who happened to land with a whaler many years before. What is interesting in this story is the fact that Roggeveen's journal makes no mention of tattoo, only body painting, yet Cook's and Forster's journal mentions the art in some detail.
[19] This plant *Cordyline frutecosa* is found throughout Polynesia.
[20] Alfred Metraux was a member of the Franco-Belgian Expedition to Easter Island in 1934/35. His book *Ethnology of Easter Island*, first published in 1940, is one of several sources on the culture of Easter Island.
[21] A *rapa* is a ceremonial dance paddle of highly stylized human form.
[22] The *komari* design is based upon the female vulva.
[23] Captain Wilhelm Geiseler of the German Imperial Navy was ordered to Easter Island at the request of the Berlin Imperial Museum in 1882 to make anthropological studies. His account was published by the University of Hawai`i in 1995 as *Geiseler's Easter Island Report; An 1880's Anthropological Account*.
[24] In a report left to us by the Spanish in 1770, they reported seeing "fearsome monstrosities," which the Rapanui called *pare*, tattooed on the abdomen of an islander.
[25] His report was later published by the National Museum in Washington in 1889.

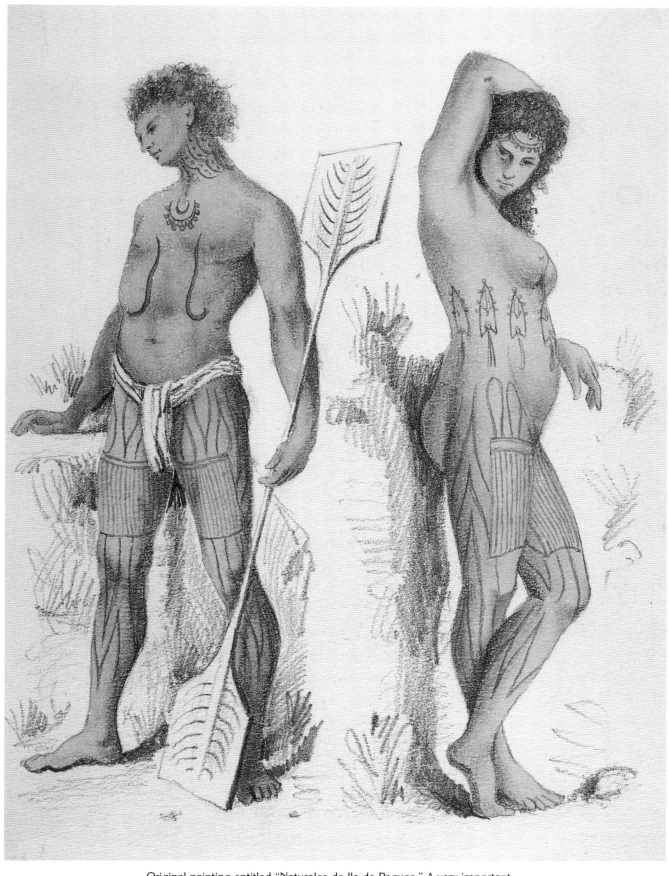

Original painting entitled "Naturales de Ile de Paques." A very important picture by Julien Viaud* painted while he was on the island in 1872. This picture shows a highly stylized representation of tattoos as observed by the young Viaud. Watercolor with pencil. Formerly in collection of Count Regley de Koenigsegg.

*Julien Viaud, alias Pierre Loti, arrived on Easter Island aboard the frigate *Le Flore* in 1872. As an aspiring naval cadet he wrote down his day-to-day impressions on this trip and many others, and used them as a basis for many of the books and poems he later wrote, the most famous being *The Marriage of Pierre Loti*.

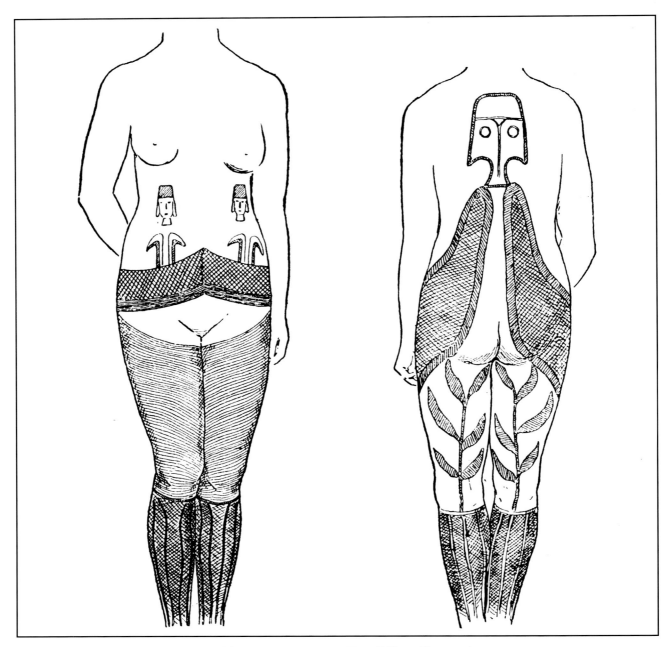

Drawing of female tattoo designs. From William Thomson's *Report of the National Museum* published in 1889. Paymaster Thomson records in this drawing a *rapa* or ceremonial dance paddle tattoo on the back and a pair of heads known as *pare pu* under the breasts. What is described as a "breeches" design appears on the legs in addition to a pattern of leaves or vines.

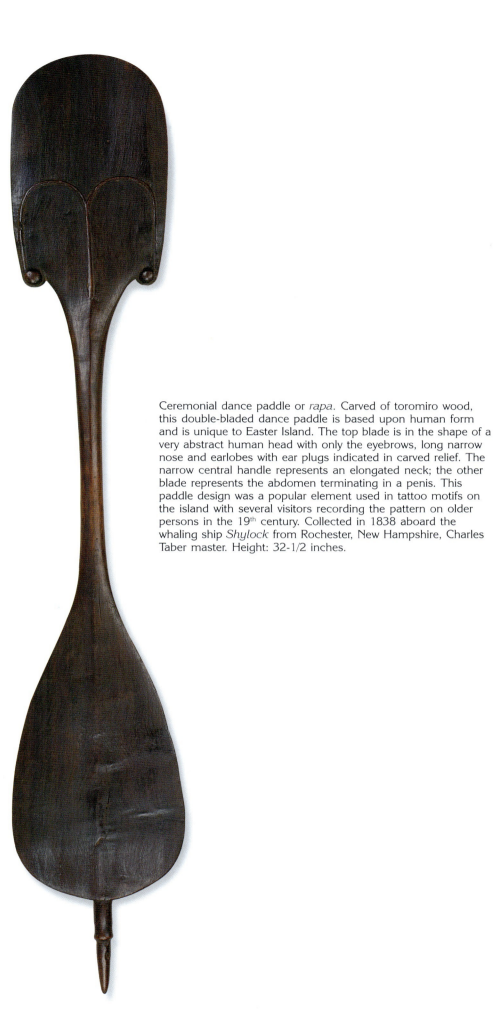

Ceremonial dance paddle or *rapa*. Carved of toromiro wood, this double-bladed dance paddle is based upon human form and is unique to Easter Island. The top blade is in the shape of a very abstract human head with only the eyebrows, long narrow nose and earlobes with ear plugs indicated in carved relief. The narrow central handle represents an elongated neck; the other blade represents the abdomen terminating in a penis. This paddle design was a popular element used in tattoo motifs on the island with several visitors recording the pattern on older persons in the 19th century. Collected in 1838 aboard the whaling ship *Shylock* from Rochester, New Hampshire, Charles Taber master. Height: 32-1/2 inches.

Drawings of male tattoo designs. These illustrations are from Hjalmar Stolpe's article* on tattooing and are good examples of facial and neck motifs. Tattooing on the forehead was known as *retu* with the series of large dots known as *humu* or *puraki*. The neck area, known as *ua*, is shown here with a tattoo of bold wavy stripes intermixed with other patterns.
*Hjalmar Stolpe's article was published in 1899 by the Zoological, Anthropological, and Ethnographical Museum in Dresden, Germany.

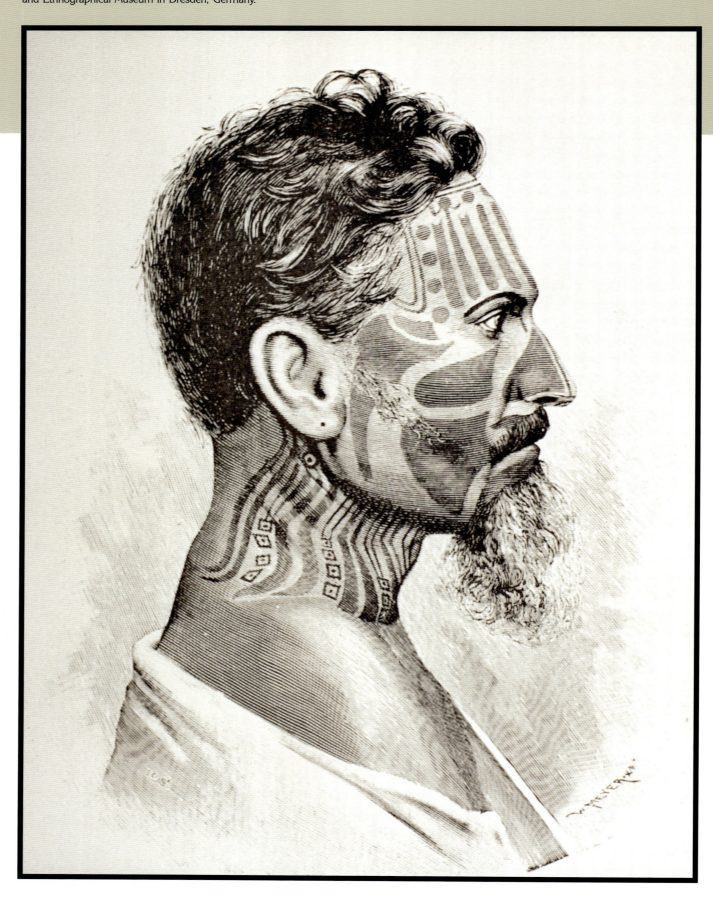

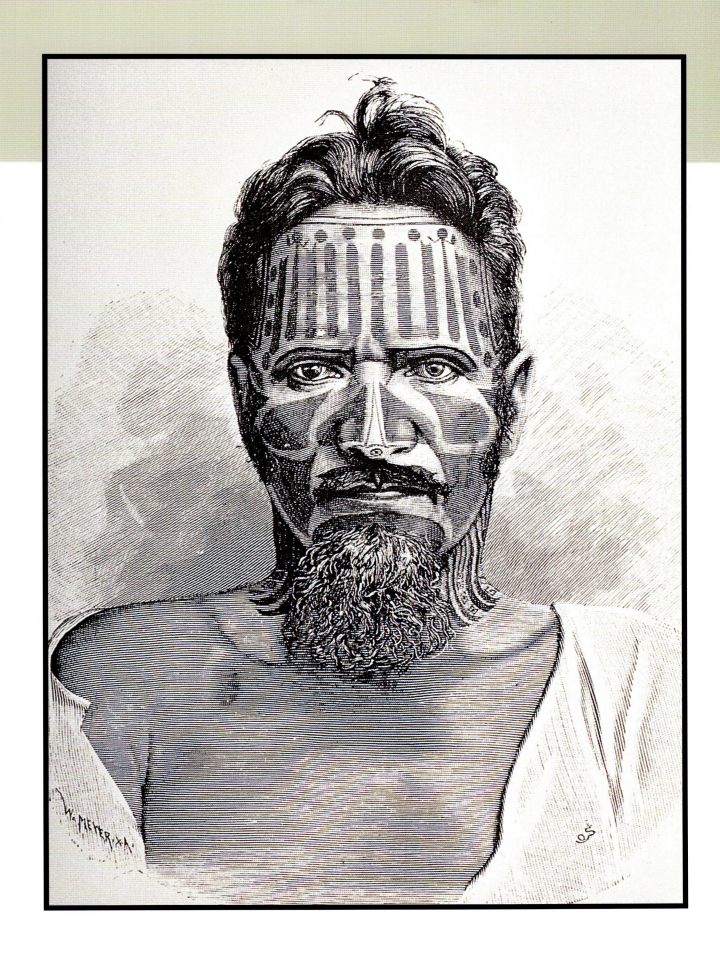

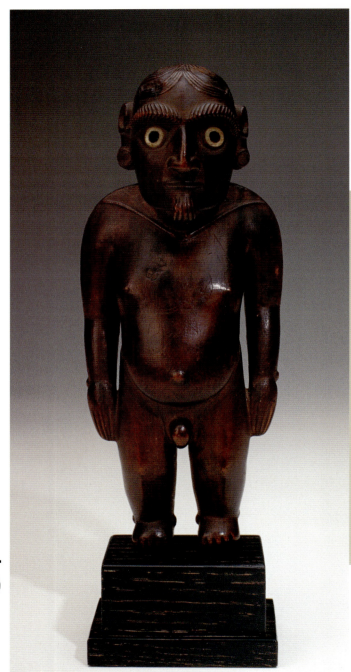
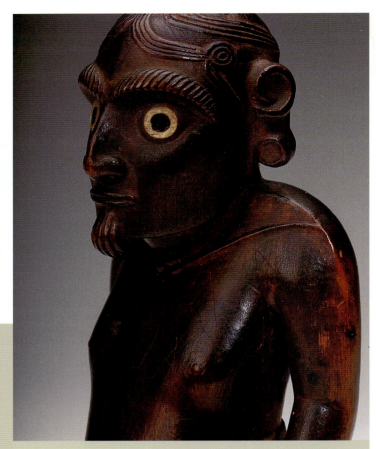

Male dwarf or child figure *moai tagnata*. Carved of toromiro wood with bird bone and obsidian eyes (one replaced with black sailcloth), this rare sculpture is most remarkable in its lifelike detail. Of an ancient type, this figure most likely represents an ancestor or mythological figure and is used in a similar fashion to the *moai kava kava*. This sculpture has a highly stylized frigate bird motif carved in relief on top its head. 18th/early 19th century. Height: 8-3/4 inches. Traces of red pigment on surface. Ex Sotheby's, New York.

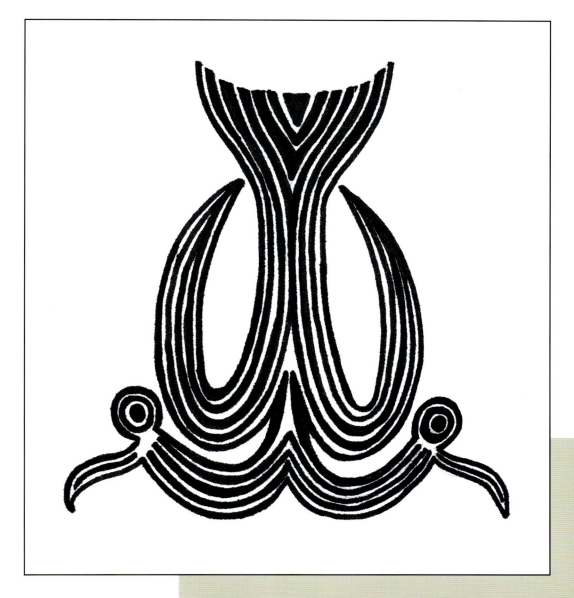

Drawing of a frigate bird motif. The glyph illustrated here is carved in relief on top of the *moai tagnata's* head. This design was seen in various forms and was tattooed on both sexes symbolizing the birdman deity, an important figure in Rapanui mythology.

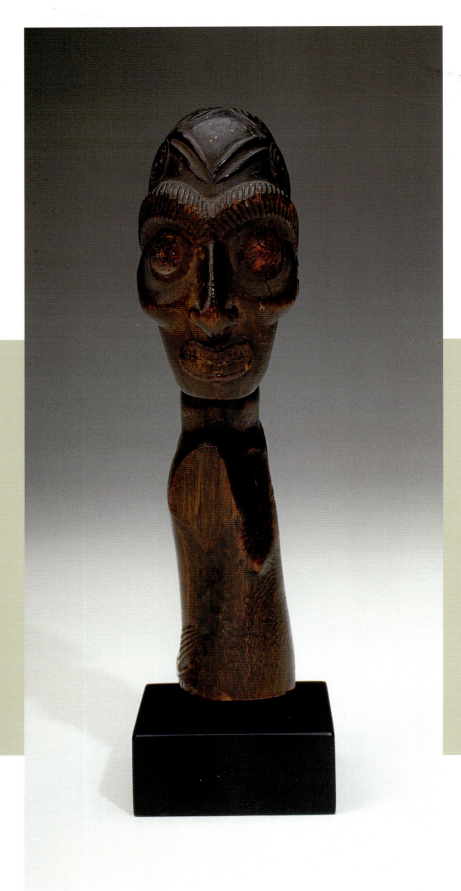

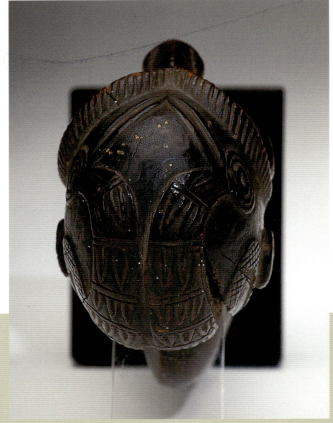

Male partial figure from a *moai tagnata*. Carved of toromiro wood with replaced eyes of red sealing wax, this partial figure has a highly realistic frigate bird glyph on its head, complete with feathers. Of an ancient type, this sculpture probably represents an ancestor figure. 18th/early 19th century. Height: 7-1/8 inches. Purchased in an old estate in Fall River, Massachusetts.

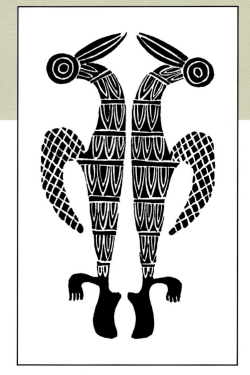

Drawing of a frigate bird motif. The glyph illustrated here is carved in relief on top of the fragmentary moai tagnata figure. This design was seen in various forms and was tattooed on both sexes symbolizing the birdman deity, an important figure in Rapa Nui mythology

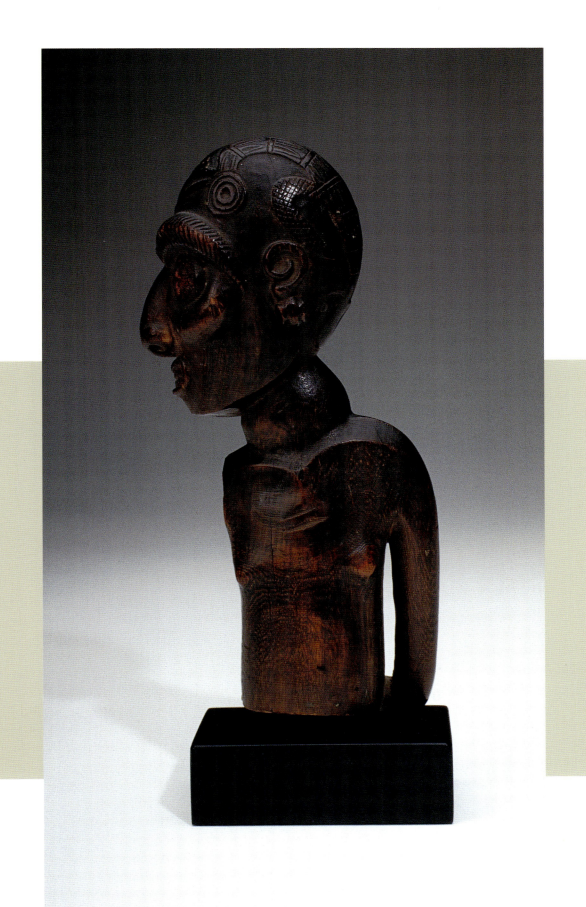

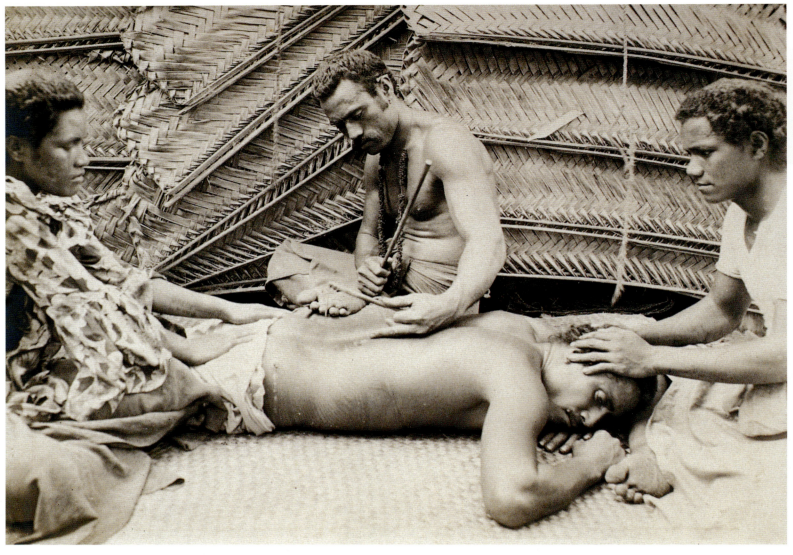

Original photograph of a man being tattooed. Reverse of the photo inscribed in pencil, Apia Samoa 1903. Gelatin silver print. Photographer unknown.

A Tattooing Artist's Song While Tattooing A Chief

Patience, only a short while, and you will see your tattoo which will resemble the fresh leaf of the ti plant.

I feel sorry for you, I wish it was a burden which I could take off your shoulders in love and carry for you.

Oh, the blood! It springs out of your body at every stroke; try to be strong.

Your necklace may break, the fau tree may burst, but my tattooing is indestructible. It is an everlasting gem that you will take into your grave.

Chorus

Oh, I am sad, you are weak, oh, I feel sorry that the pain follows you even in your sleep and you resist it.

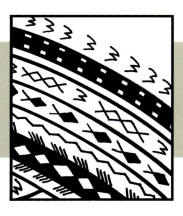

SAMOA

The word Samoa is used here to describe the entire group of Samoan Islands comprising present-day American Samoa and Western Samoa. Forming a chain, the islands lie approximately 1,200 miles west-north-west/east-southeast of Tahiti and only 300 miles north-northeast of Tonga. The main islands are Savai'i and Upolu in Western Samoa and Tutuila in American Samoa. All the islands are of volcanic origin with the exception of tiny Rose atoll in the American group. On the island of Savai'i volcanic slopes rise to over 6,000 feet with dramatic scenery.

Due to the proximity to the equator, all of the islands enjoy a warm tropical climate. Hurricanes occasionally occur in the summer months, sometimes with devastating results. Because of its warm climate, the vegetation is extremely lush in most areas and coastal lowlands are rich and fertile, offering easy cultivation of crops such as yams, breadfruits and sweet potatoes.

Archaeological excavations have revealed very early dates of occupation. Recent carbon dating has put settlement between 2500 and 300 BC, in line with somewhat similar dates from neighboring Fiji and Tonga. All three of these groups seem to have been inhabited by similar people, often referred to as *Lapita,* and appear to be the original colonists to Central and East Polynesia. There is evidence in both oral traditions as well as archaeologically that between 1200 and 1600 AD the group was occupied by Tongans. This long period of contact by Tongans led to considerable intermixture and accounts for many similarities between the two cultures. Finally around 1600 AD the Tongans were expelled, but even to the present day much intermarriage and contact has gone on between the two cultures.

The first European to discover Samoa was the Dutch explorer Roggeveen who sighted Manu'a, where he briefly engaged in trading in 1722. It was the next European, the French explorer Bougainville, who gave the group the name "Navigator Islands"[1] when he sighted the islands in 1768. Bougainville did not land on the islands but noted in his journals the great skills of the native canoeist. Throughout the rest of the 18th and early 19th centuries the usual assortment of whalers and traders briefly made landfall in the islands, but it was not until 1830 that a permanent European presence was in place with the London Missionary Society[2] station at Upolu. By the 1840s Christianity was firmly in place due to the work of this London-based group.[3]

During this time of European intervention in the islands, Malietoa Vaiinupo came into power and was termed "king" by the local authorities. It was Malietoa - whose family who had been most instrumental in expelling the Tongans - who established control over the whole island chain. In a complicated series of events, Great Britain, Germany and the United States intervened in local politics and disputes - some among themselves - leading to the group being divided in 1889. The group was split into two areas: The one administered by Germany was comprised of Western Samoa (Savai'i and Upolu); the United States administered the eastern islands from Pago Pago[4] on Tutuila in present-day American Samoa. In 1914 at the start of World War One, New Zealand occupied Western Samoa with their expeditionary forces and, in 1920 under a mandate from the League of Nations, the islands continued under their control until 1962, at which time independence was fully granted.

As on many Polynesian islands, Samoan society was and still is a stratified affair based upon rank and title, all according to birth and position within one's family. It is chiefs or *ali'i* and their assistants, known as talking chiefs or *tulafale,* that claim descent from divine ancestors. The heads of families are titleholders and are eligible for participation in village councils or *fonos*. These village councils are responsible to larger district assemblies, which are under control of the most powerful chief.

One of the more unusual aspects of Samoan society was the honoring of a virgin in each village with a title. These females known as *taupou* usually were the eldest niece or daughter of the village chief. Holding the second highest position in the village, her duties were mainly ceremonial. Described by the noted anthropologist Margaret Mead[5] as the "female ornament of the chiefs rank," they would be dressed in ornate costumes on these special occasions.

As in all areas of Polynesia, *tapu* was ever-present, being reflected in the divine ancestry of chiefs where it was associated with their person or personal belongings. These *tapu* regulations were as elaborate in Samoa as they were with the chiefs of closely related Tonga and Hawai`i, where there are quite a few similarities.

Samoan spear or *tao*. Spears like this were chiefly weapons and ornately carved with a series of complex barbs and projections. The design elements used in this type of spear relate very closely to some tattoo motifs. Patterns based on fishing spear barbs, which are somewhat similar, were known as *fa'aulutao*. Length: 37 inches. Early 19th century.

The gods or *atua* in Samoa were somewhat more limited than other areas of East Polynesia with *Tangaloa* being the most important deity. He was the sky god and was seen in Samoan society as the creator of the world and humankind. Spirits of deified chiefs were as known *tupua*, with *aitu* the general term for minor gods associated with domestic affairs.

Samoan households were grouped in scattered villages mainly along the coasts of the islands. Basically consisting of one-room dwellings, these *fale'o'o* were accompanied by a cooking house with other associated buildings consisting of communal guest and ceremonial houses.

Vegetable foodstuffs in the group consisted primarily of taro or *talo* and coconut or *niu*; these were supplemented by breadfruits, yams and sweet potatoes. On ceremonial occasions pig or *pua'a* was served, but fish, so abundant in local waters, was the main source of day-to-day non-vegetable food.

Artistic pursuits were varied in the islands, with the title of *tufunga* given to respected craftsmen whose services were exchanged for food and hospitality. Their duties were many, consisting of the skilled manufacture of canoes, houses and the like. Women's pursuits were concerned with the making of *siapo* or barkcloth along with the fiber arts, consisting of mat making, some of these mats being an important commodity in ceremonial gift exchanges.[6]

The art of tattoo or *tatau* was practiced on both sexes and was a mark of adulthood as well as ornamentation. Ti-leaf-plaited kilts or *titi* were the usual daily wear, with people of rank wearing either barkcloth kilts or *lavalava* as well as mats constructed of finely woven pandanus leaf.

War was frequently waged, and Samoans were well known for their fighting ability, with major campaigns fought against frequent Tongan incursions. Besides these events, Samoans often fought among themselves, avenging personal insults or in revenge occasioned by a military defeat. War clubs of many different types and forms were used in close combat with severely contested battles fought in open situations. Often these clubs were obtained in trade with the neighboring islands of Tonga and Fiji. Spears or *tao* were also used and were popular and effective weapons of choice with complex barbs and projections. With the advent of the missionaries in 1830 these skirmishes greatly diminished.

Towards the end of the 19th century Samoa had its fair share of famous and infamous Europeans. The most famous of these, the noted Scottish author Robert Louis Stevenson,[7] arrived in Samoa with his entourage in 1889. Suffering from years of tuberculosis, he found the group's climate the only place in the world where he could lead something of a normal life, free from the severe hemorrhages that had plagued him for so long. Here he built a house on a forested hill called Vailima, where he provided regal-style feasts for both chiefs and European visitors alike. Served by natives dressed in Royal Stewart tartan *lavala*, they provided a source of relief for this chief of the Vailima clan. It was at Vailima where he first expressed in his letters a strong affection for the Polynesian people calling them "God's best, at least God's sweetest work." Stevenson died on his veranda in 1894 suffering a massive stroke. It seemed only fitting that after his death Samoans made a road in tribute from the capital Apia to Vailima, where his house eventually became Government House.

In spite of years of considerable foreign contact, there has not been a total rejection of Samoan traditional culture, the people being far more resistant to change than many other Polynesians. This has resulted in the culture basically intact, although heavily influenced by various forms of Christianity. In an interesting twist of fate, like neighboring Tonga, the group's largest export today is its people, who have, in the case of Western Samoa, emmigrated to neighboring New Zealand.[69] In American Samoa, like its counterpart, there has been a great exodus of Samoans to cities in the United States, with Honolulu, Los Angeles, Seattle, Reno and Las Vegas all being the main metropolitan areas of choice. Whether or not the culture can remain intact with these migrations, only time will tell.

Samoan Tattooing - *tatau*

Samoan tattooing or *tatau* was done on both men and women. The men were extensively tattooed from the waist to the knee and occasionally on the hands. Tattooing of women, on the other hand, rarely extended beyond the upper thighs, with the majority of the tattooing limited to the area from the waist to the genitals and occasionally behind the knees. Women's hands and wrists also often were tattooed giving a pleasing affect.

Like other areas in Polynesia the tattooing consisted of pricking the skin with a tattooing comb or *au*. This comb was constructed of turtle shell or bone plates. Neatly bound with coir fibers onto a haft of light *fau* wood, the comb then would be dipped into a pigment composed of candlenut (*Aleurites Moluccana*) soot and water. The comb then was tapped into the skin with a mallet or *sausau* traditionally made from a piece of coconut-leaflet midrib or wood, thus creating a pattern of mainly rectilinear design elements.

The tattoo artist who applied the tattoo was known as the *tufuga tatau*, spending many years mastering the art. To practice he would spend hours and sometimes days tapping designs into sand or barkcloth. The act of tattooing was a solemn affair, with the tattooing of a chief's son a celebration for the whole village.

Obtaining a tattoo was and still is a great challenge. A sacred aspect of Samoan culture, it is a permanent mark showing both endurance as well as dedication. It has been said that the *tatau* purifies the soul and gives one a new perception of life. Its strength lies in the beauty and pride the wearer enjoys. The process was not without risk, with the onset of an infection a very real possibility. This often resulted in the death of the participant.[9]

Due to the great pain involved in the tattooing process a person often could not endure the suffering, ending the operation in midstream. For the rest of his life this person hence would be subjected to a great deal of ridicule and embarrassment. Traditionally all men, with almost no exception, subjected themselves to obtaining tattoos at the onset of puberty. Those who did not were called *pala'ai* or cowards. It was said that the women especially despised these men and that chiefs refused to accept food from their hands calling them "stinking."[10] Acquiring a tattoo was so important that during the last century many young people who were being prepared for mission service often turned their backs on the mission schools, the only reason being that they were forbidden from being tattooed. This has changed somewhat at the present time as many religious leaders today realize the importance of tattoo in Samoan society.

Tattooing was often a ceremonial affair and in the case of a young chief a very elaborate one. Early observers recorded that the ceremony was usually opened with sham fights and war exercises. Before beginning the actual procedure a distribution of gifts to the *tufuga* would be made. Consisting of fine mats and other precious heirlooms, these gifts were highly valued and are today more valuable than money.[11]

The actual process of tattooing consisted of the *tufuga* handling the instruments while others held down the participant and tightened the skin. The comb was then dipped into the pigment and placed upon the skin. The mallet then struck the comb, driving the sharp edges into the flesh, repeating this until the designs were complete. In the case of men, the pattern to be carried out first was the *tua* stripe, which extended over the whole back. The operation lasted until dusk or until the participant could withstand the pain no longer. Early the next morning the operation would start all over again until finished. At times, however, the artist would have to interrupt his work for several days to let the inflammation heal. It could take up to three months for a complete tattoo to be finished, depending on the person's stamina. The last design to be completed would then be placed over the navel. Feasting would begin with family members and supporters helping the person stand proud in his pain. Final gifts were then presented to the *tufuga* in a solemn ceremony, with a water vessel smashed at the tattooed person's feet marking the end of the ordeal. The whole act and festivities over, a sprinkling of the tattooed with coconut milk would now make the tattoos touchable by others.

With the entire process finished, the healing began, which involved a complex process of soaking the body in seawater for many hours at a time with the flesh constantly being massaged to work out all the impurities. This was done with the assistance of friends and family, as the tattooed areas were greatly inflamed. Simple tasks like walking and sitting were impossible to do alone. Design elements in the tattoo would take five to six months to distinctly appear on the body and nearly a year to completely heal.

The area of tattooing on women was much smaller than that of men with the majority of the tattoos being of the *punialo* form. This form of tattoo, which was said to be particularly attractive to the opposite sex, was done on the abdomen between the umbilicus and the genitals. This was the only type of tattoo that extended beyond the thighs, the majority being limited from the genitals to the knees. The most common tattoo seen on women was the *malu* and covered only the hollows of the knees and their immediate surroundings. Hand tattoos were a common occurrence, being done on young girls at the same time of the tattooing of a young chief.[12] It was said that only women with this hand tattoo or *lima* could prepare and serve *kava*[75] on ceremonial occasions. Tattooing of common people was always carried out in a much less careful manner than those persons of high rank. Early observers remarked at the considerable difference in the quality of workmanship between the two.

Tattooing in Samoa still lives on today, having never fully been extinguished by overzealous missionaries. The *mana* of the person, like in the past, is further enhanced by the wearing of his or her *tatau*, adding to the essential underlying elements of Samoan society. The *tatau* thus encompasses all things Samoan.

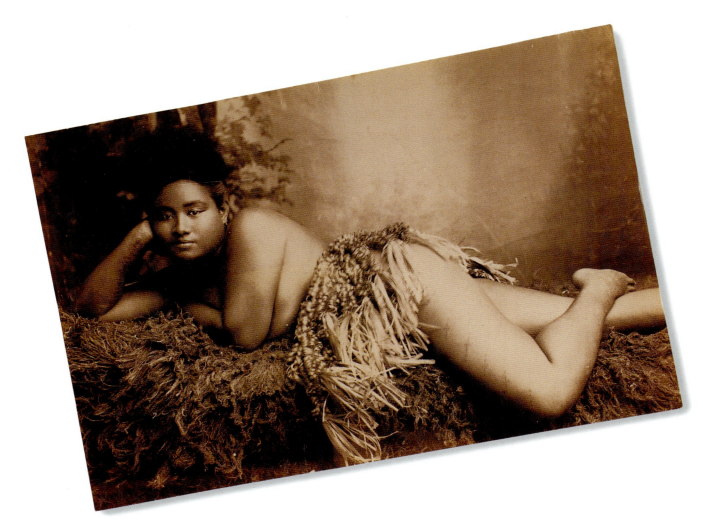

Original photograph of reclining woman. This studio portrait shows what appear to be *vae'ali* patterns on the legs. This albumen photograph, with penciled inscription "J.Davis" on reverse, more likely is the work of photographer Thomas Andrew.* Semi-erotic photographs like the one shown here were very popular during the age of prudish Victorian values.

*John Davis (? –1893) was producing photographs as early as 1870 in his Apia studio for the souvenir trade. His studio also acted as the local post office with Davis as postmaster. His most famous product was a series of Christmas cards of Samoan subject matter, which he made for the local market. Following his death, A.J. Tattersall acquired his negatives continuing to print and sell them for many years.

Translation of Design Names According to Marquardt

alu'alu	jellyfish
anufe	caterpillar or worm
'aso	stripes, based upon rafters of Samoan houses
'asofa'aifo	serrated stripes, based upon rafters of the roof of a Samoan house running down from its top in the same patterns as the 'asofa'aifo stripes
'aso o le fusi	pattern forming the fusi band in the hollow of the knee. The short stripes of the design in their combination resemble the rafters of the roof.
'asotalitu	overall name of the tattoo changes in the place where it is found/to be gone
atigivae	nail on the foot/claw on the foot
aveau	starfish
fa'aatualoa	centipede
fa'aila	birthmark
fa'amuli'ali'ao	pointed triangular pattern named after the pointed end of a type of shellfish
fa'atalalaupaogo	spiny leaf of the pandanus tree
fa'aulutao	fishing spear
fa'a'upega	net used for catching fish and birds
fa'avala	lavalava or loin cloth/or flesh parts left open
fetu	star
fusi	band/belt
gogo	seabird
ivimutu	endbone
lausae	meaning unknown
malu	protection/shadow
pula	yellow taro root
pulatama	child/offspring
punialo	enclosed place for fishing/hide or conceal
pute	navel
saimutu	meaning unknown, but the stripes are of great importance as they are an identification of the ancestry of the bearer
selu	hair comb
tafani	name of a portion of tattooing
tapulu	having to do with restriction/forbidden
tasele	fast beating/to make part of the tattoo
togitogi	to mark a part of the tattoo
toluse	cross/based upon the cross-like design in the jellyfish, not the cross in Christianity – and considered a very old design
tua	back
ulumanu	bird head
vae'ali	headrest feet

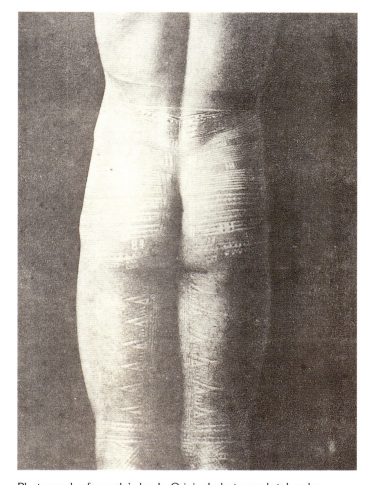

Photograph of a male's back. Original photograph taken by Carl Marquardt in Samoa sometime in the 1890s and later published in his book *The Tattooing of Both Sexes in Samoa*, published in Berlin in 1899.

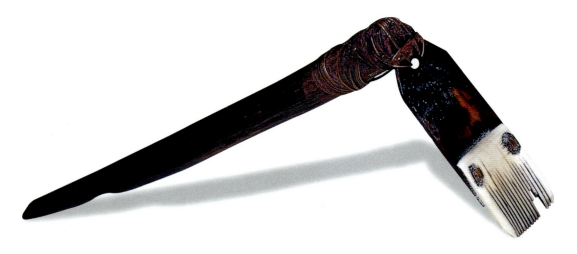

Tattooing needle or comb. Termed *au*, this example has a turtle shell plate. Length: 6-5/8 inches. 19th century. Ex collection of Leo Fortess.

Endnotes

[1] The name Navigator Islands was a term used for the present-day Samoan group of islands. This name was used well into the 19th century.

[2] The London Missionary Society station was manned by both Tahitian and English missionaries after the first visit of the Reverend John Williams, who was the first person to describe tattooing in Samoa with the brief statement: "Few of the women were tattooed but many of them were spotted." His published account, *A Narrative of Missionary Enterprises in the South Sea Islands*, published in London in 1830, totally ignores tattooing of men; why this was done is anyone's guess.

[3] A detailed account of Samoan culture before the arrival of Christianity was left by the London Missionary Reverend George Turner who published his accounts in 1861 in the book entitled *Nineteen Years in Polynesia: Missionary Life, Travel and Researches*.

[4] The port of Pago Pago (pronounced Pango Pango) became an important United States naval base with a major coaling station set up. The United States administers American Samoa today and is a U.S. Trust Territory.

[5] Noted anthropologist Margaret Mead's (1901-1978) landmark book on Samoa was entitled *Coming of Age in Samoa*. Published in 1930, it was based on her fieldwork in Ta'u, American Samoa in 1925-26. Mead's perception of the Samoan culture as a paradise without rape, aggression or sexual guilt has been widely disputed. Many people, especially those in the academic community, see her supporting the stereotype of a Polynesian utopia.

[6] Barkcloth and fine mats are important parts of ceremonial gift-giving even to this day. The author witnessed one gift of fine mats presented to the King of Tonga on occasion of his 80th birthday. In that presentation over 800 fine mats were given by the Samoan delegation to the King on July 4, 1998.

[7] Robert Louis Stevenson (1850-1894), known by the Samoans as *Tusitalia* or "teller of tales," arrived on his yacht *Casco* accompanied by his American stepson and literary collaborator Lloyd Osbourne, along with Stevenson's mother, his wife Fanny, Joseph Strong - who was the official court painter to King Kalakaua of Hawai`i - and Belle, who was Stevenson's stepdaughter and wife of the painter Strong. Stevenson wrote many South Pacific tales including *In the South Seas* and *The Bottle Imp*, which - in his own estimation -"was one of my best works."

[8] Auckland, New Zealand, now contains the largest population in the world of Polynesian people located in one metropolitan area. The Polynesian population consists of Samoans, Tongans, Niueans, Cook Islanders and Maori peoples.

[9] It has been reported that currently in Western Samoa the pigment or dye used in tattooing is rust collected in discarded tin cans mixed with candlenut soot and water. The author knows of one case in particular where a European obtained a partial leg tattoo using this concoction for the tattooer's ink that resulted in the legs swelling twice their normal size, accompanied by a high fever and excruciating pain. It was only with antibiotics that the person brought with him from Honolulu that enabled him to survive. Needless to say he did not complete his full tattoo.

[10] This according to Carl Marquardt in his book entitled *The Tattooing of both sexes in Samoa*, published in Berlin in 1899. He went on further to state: "I sometimes had the opportunity to observe that untattooed men wear their lavalava especially far down in order to deceive the observer on their shortcomings."

[11] These heirlooms or *measina ale atunu'u* are articles that have been within the family for several generations, in the process acquiring much *mana* and prestige.

[12] This according to Carl Marquardt in his book entitled *The Tattooing of both sexes in Samoa*, published in Berlin in 1899.

[13] *Kava* was prepared from the root of the *Piper methysticum* plant. Served in liquid form mixed with water, it played an integral part in all ceremonial occasions. A mild narcotic, it is now accepted by Western medicine for its wide range of benefits. It produces a mild euphoric effect.

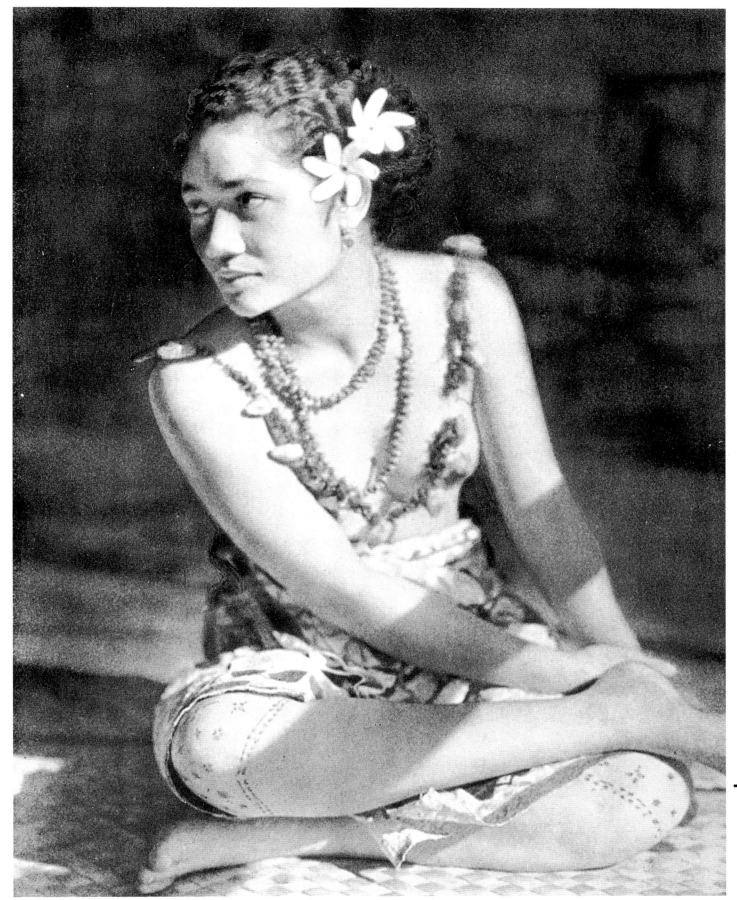

Photograph of a *taupou*. Photographed by Frances Hubbard Flaherty in Safune, Savai'i, in 1923. Originally published in the magazine *Asia* in an article by her entitled "Setting up House and Shop in Samoa: The Struggle to Find Screen Material in the Lyric Beauty of Polynesian Life," August 1925. Her caption of photo reads as follows: "Easily recognizable is the Samoan "taupou", the most lovely of village maidens, who is carefully guarded and then married at the appointed time by the chiefs of her village to some neighboring chief. On ceremonious occasions the taupou dresses in old Samoan style, wearing nothing but necklaces above the waist." Her tattoos appear to be of a combination of styles with traces of the *aveau* design present.

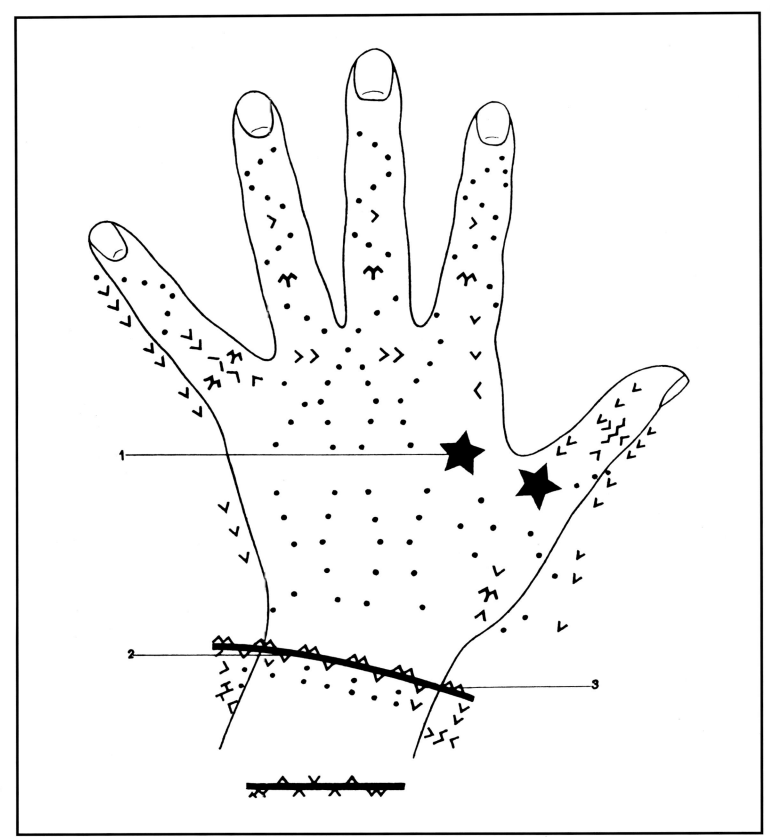

Drawing of female hand tattoos. This illustration is accompanied by pattern names in Samoan as recorded by Carl Marquardt.
1. fetu
2. fusi
3. fa'amuli'ali'ao

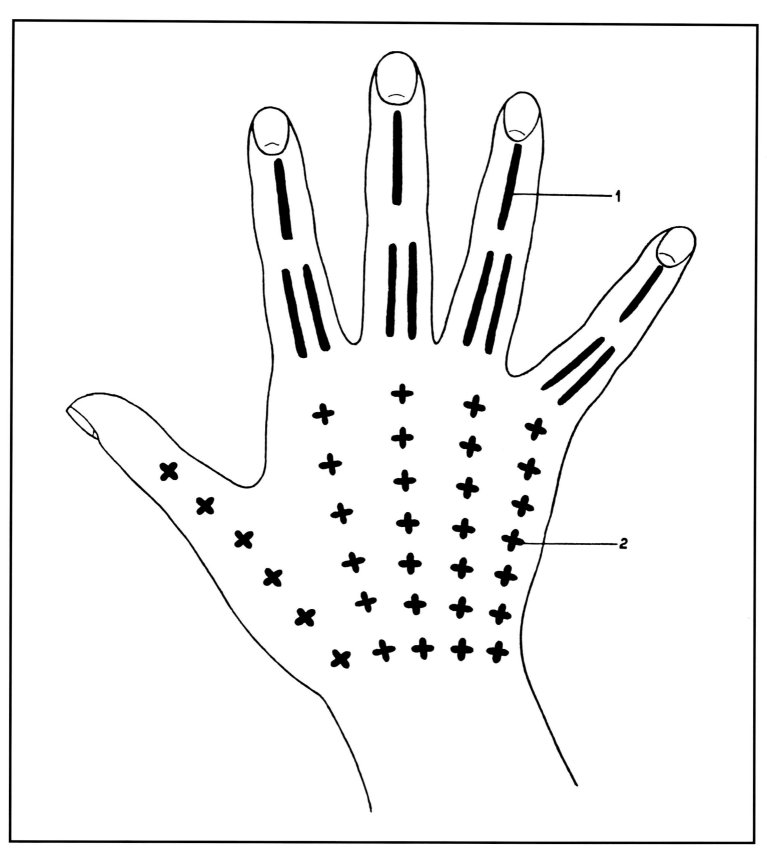

Drawing of female hand tattoos. This illustration is accompanied by pattern names in Samoan as recorded by Carl Marquardt.
1. anufe
2. fetu

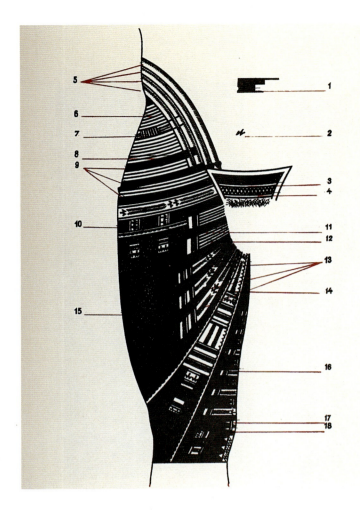

Drawing of male tattoo designs, front view. This illustration is accompanied by the pattern names in Samoan as recorded by Carl Marquardt.
1. pute
2. gogo
3. tapulu
4. fa'a'upega
5. 'asofa'aifo
6. 'aso
7. tafani
8. fa'aila
9. saimutu
10. 'assotalitu
11. fa'atalaiaupaogo
12. selu
13. fa'avala
14. fa'aatualoa
15. tapulu
16. fa'atalalaupaogo
17. fusi
18. ulumanu

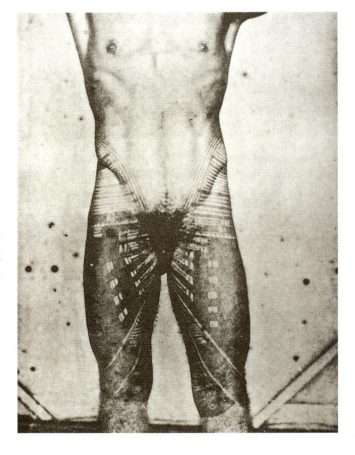

Photograph of a male's front side. Original photograph taken by Carl Marquardt in Samoa sometime in the 1890s and later published in his book *The Tattooing of Both Sexes in Samoa*, published in Berlin in 1899.

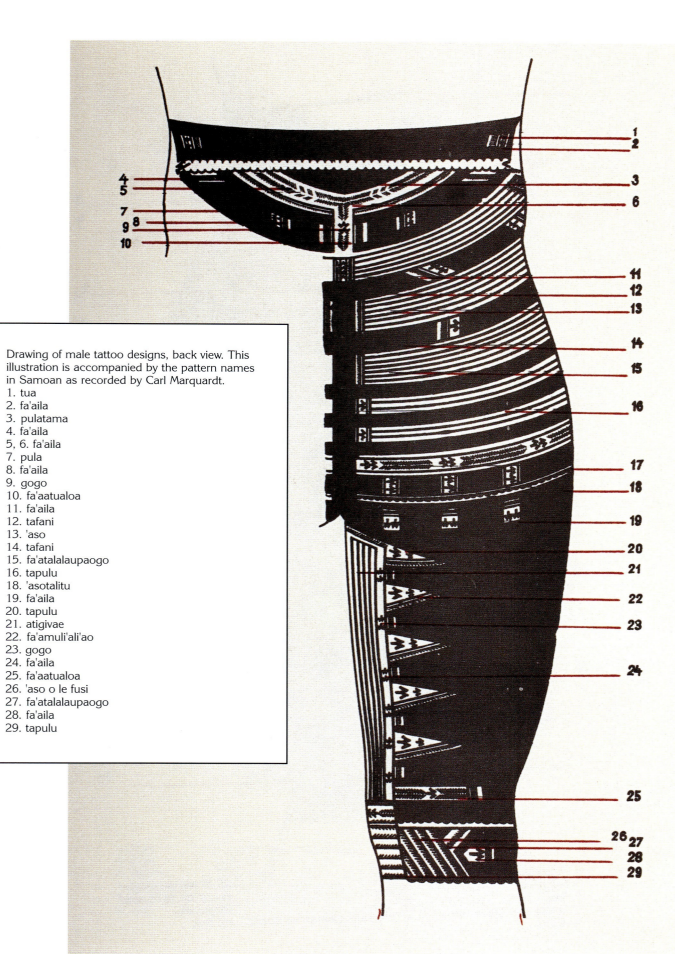

Drawing of male tattoo designs, back view. This illustration is accompanied by the pattern names in Samoan as recorded by Carl Marquardt.
1. tua
2. fa'aila
3. pulatama
4. fa'aila
5, 6. fa'aila
7. pula
8. fa'aila
9. gogo
10. fa'aatualoa
11. fa'aila
12. tafani
13. 'aso
14. tafani
15. fa'atalalaupaogo
16. tapulu
18. 'asotalitu
19. fa'aila
20. tapulu
21. atigivae
22. fa'amuli'ali'ao
23. gogo
24. fa'aila
25. fa'aatualoa
26. 'aso o le fusi
27. fa'atalalaupaogo
28. fa'aila
29. tapulu

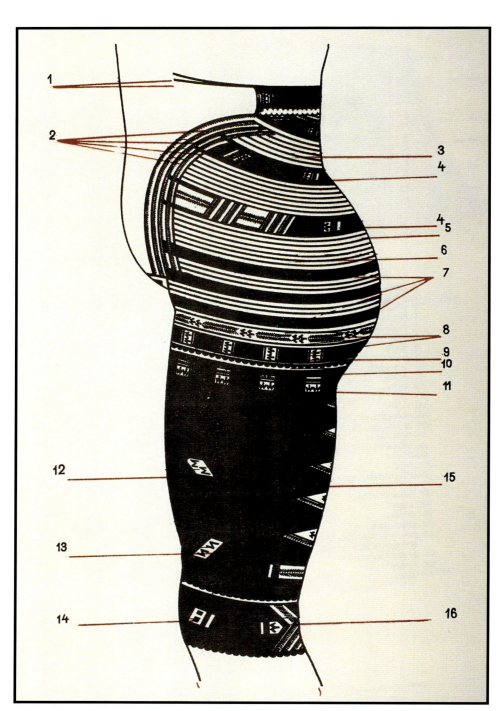

Drawing of male tattoo designs, side view. This illustration is accompanied by the pattern names in Samoan as recorded by Carl Marquardt.
1. fa'aulutao
2. 'asofa'aifo
3. 'aso
4. tafani
5. fa'aila
6. 'aso
7. aaimutu
8. 'aso
9. 'asostalitu
10. fa'atalalaupaogo
11,12,13,14. fa'aila
15. tapulu
16. fusi

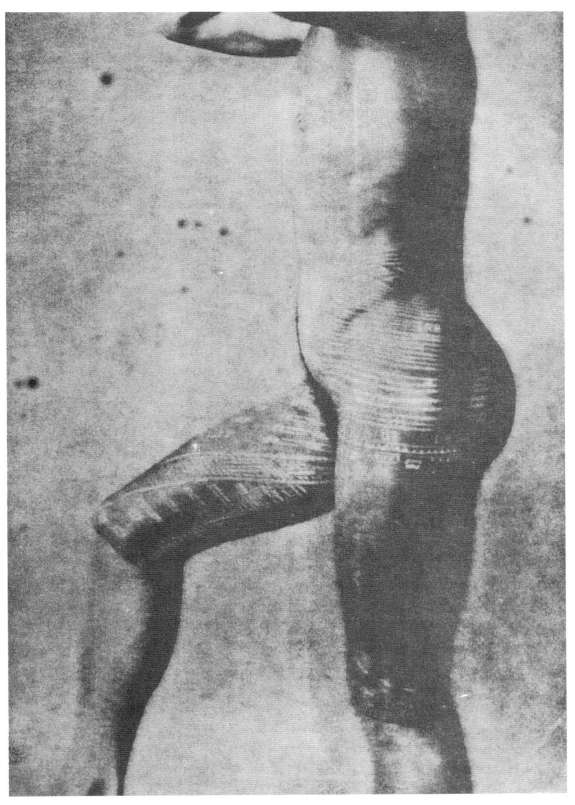

Photograph of a side view of a male. Original photograph taken by Carl Marquardt in Samoa sometime in the 1890s and later published in his book *The Tattooing of Both Sexes in Samoa*, published in Berlin in 1899.

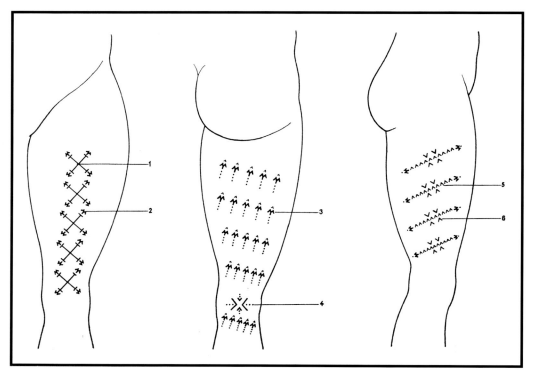

Drawing of female tattoo designs: Front, back, and outer side views. This illustration is accompanied by the pattern names in Samoan as recorded by Carl Marquardt.
1. toluse
2, 3. gogo
4. malu
5, 6. vae'ali

Drawing of female tattoo designs: Front, back, and outer side views. This illustration is accompanied by the pattern names in Samoan as recorded by Carl Marquardt.
1. toluse
2. anufe
3. 'alu'alu
4. malu
5. anufe
6. 'alu'alu

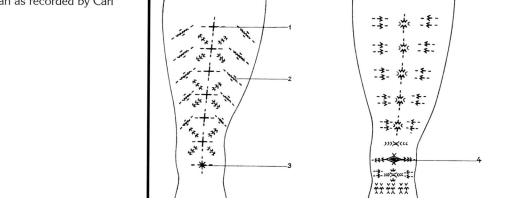

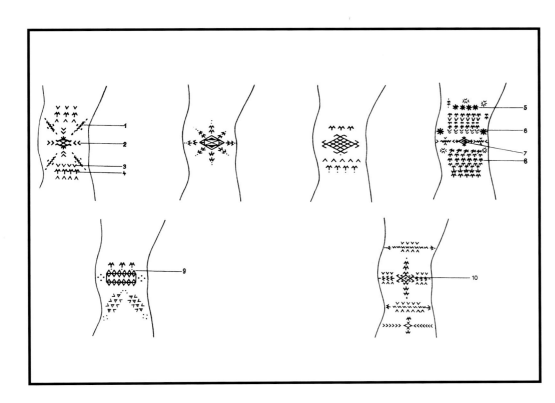

Drawing of female tattoo designs located in the hollows of the knees. Women with this type of tattoo, known as *malu*, were only tattooed in this one area, according to Carl Marquardt.
1. anufe
2, 3. vae'ali
4. gogo
5. 'alu'alu
6. vae'ali
7. malu
8. gogo
9. fa'amuli'ali'ao
10. malu

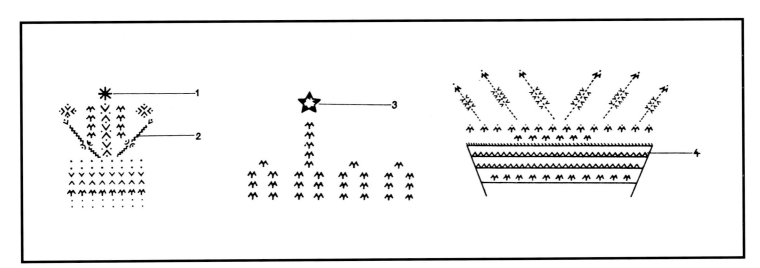

Drawing of female *punialo* tattoo designs. This type of pattern is found in both sexes and is located between the navel and pubic area. The center design according to Carl Marquardt was recorded on a girl of royal ancestry.
1. 'alu'alu
2. anufe
3. fetu
4. fa'amuli'ali'ao

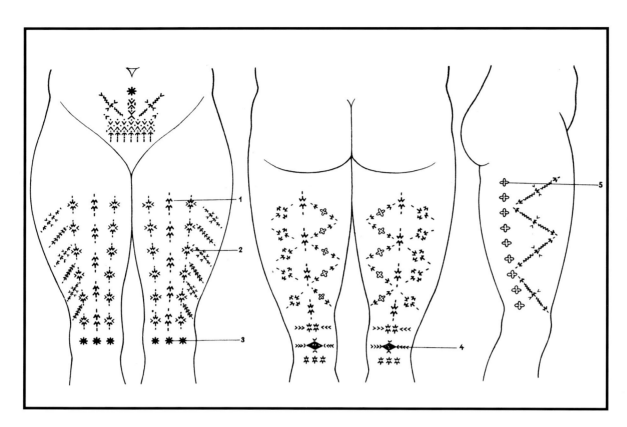

Drawing of female tattoo designs: front, back and outer side views. This illustration is accompanied by the pattern names in Samoan as recorded by Carl Marquardt.
1. gogo
2. vae'ali
3. 'alu'alu
4. malu
5. fetu

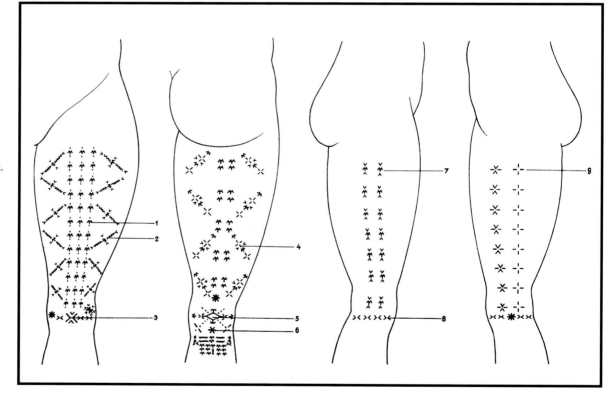

Drawing of female tattoo designs: Front, back, outer side and inner side views. This illustration is accompanied by the pattern names in Samoan as recorded by Carl Marquardt.
1. gogo
2. anufe
3. vae'ali
4. aveau
5. malu
6. 'alu'alu
7. gogo
8. vae'ali
9. aveau

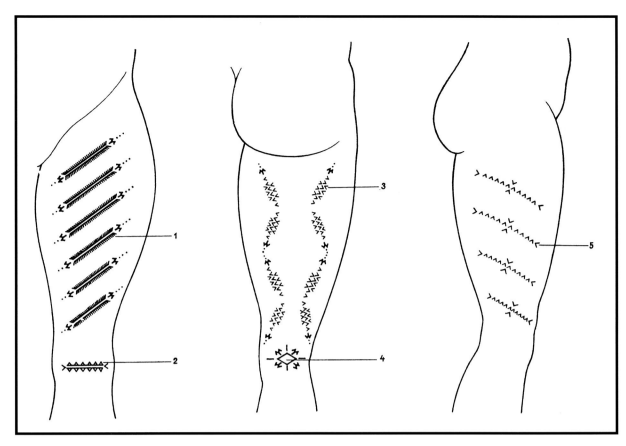

Drawing of female tattoo designs: Front, back, and outer side views. This illustration is accompanied by the pattern names in Samoan as recorded by Carl Marquardt.
1. fa'aatualoa
2. fa'amuli'ali'ao
3. vae'ali
4. malu
5. vae'ali

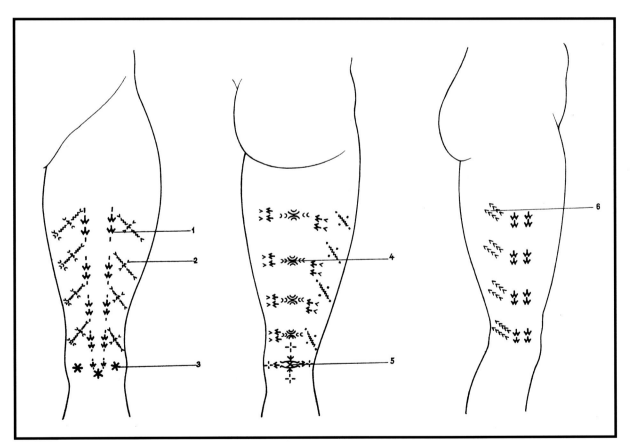

Drawing of female tattoo designs: Front, back, and outer side views. This illustration is accompanied by the pattern names in Samoan as recorded by Carl Marquardt.
1. gogo
2. vae'ali
3. 'alu'alu
4. vae'ali
5. malu
6. vae'ali

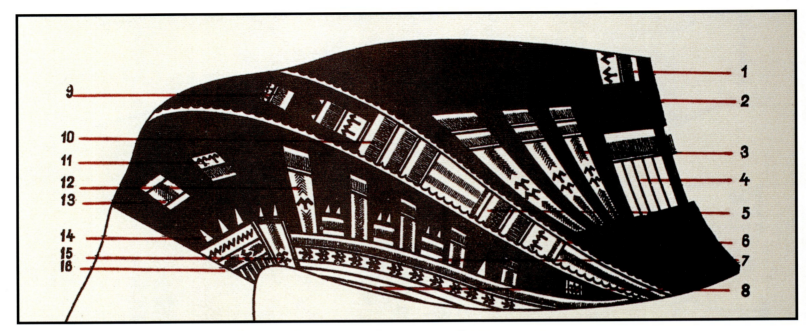

Drawing of male tattoo designs, inner leg. This illustration is accompanied by the pattern names in Samoan as recorded by Carl Marquardt.
1. fa'aila
2. tapulu
3. fa'avala
4. selu
5. fusi
6. tapulu
7. fa'aila
8. atigivae
9. fa'aila
10. fa'atalalaupaogo
11, 12, 13. fa'aila
14. fa'amuli'ali'ao
15, 16. fa'aila

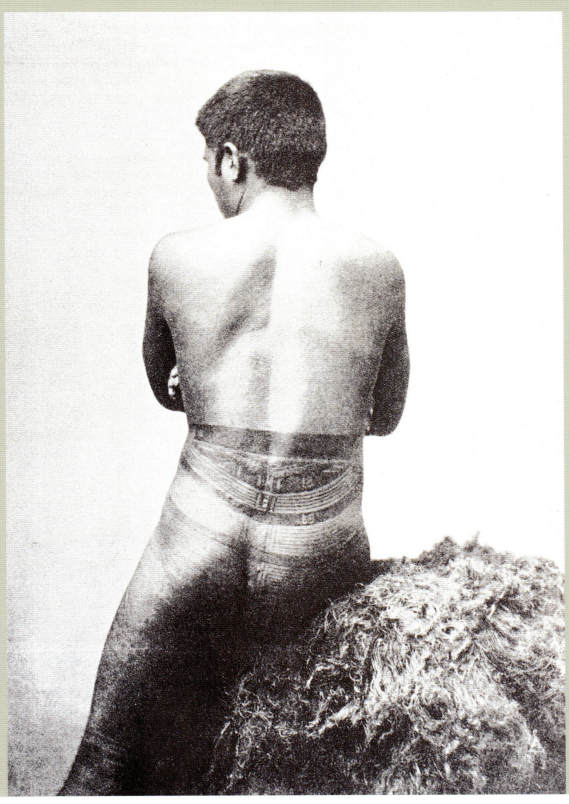

Photograph of a man from behind. This photograph was acquired by Dr. Augustin Friedrich Kramer* during one of his many trips to the Pacific in the latter part of the 19th century. This image shows the various patterns used in a man's tattoo on the backside. Albumen photograph taken by Thomas Andrew** around 1893.

*Dr. Augustin Friedrich Kramer (1865-1941) was a surgeon in the German Imperial Navy. He traveled widely and was a well-known ethnographer, publishing several books including a two-volume set on Samoa. Published in 1903 and entitled *Die Samoa Insel*, it is considered a classic on the subject. In Hawai`i, he became so dispirited with the state of the native population that he resolved to abandon his formal training in the sciences and record Samoa's life and culture before it was too late, hence the aforementioned book.

**Thomas Andrew (1855-1939) opened a studio in Apia immediately after his arrival in Samoa in 1891, and by 1899 was the owner of a thriving rubber and coconut plantation. He produced a wide range of photographs like his contemporary John Davis. His photographs, intended for the souvenir market, are marked by a sense of dignity and composure not often found during this time period.

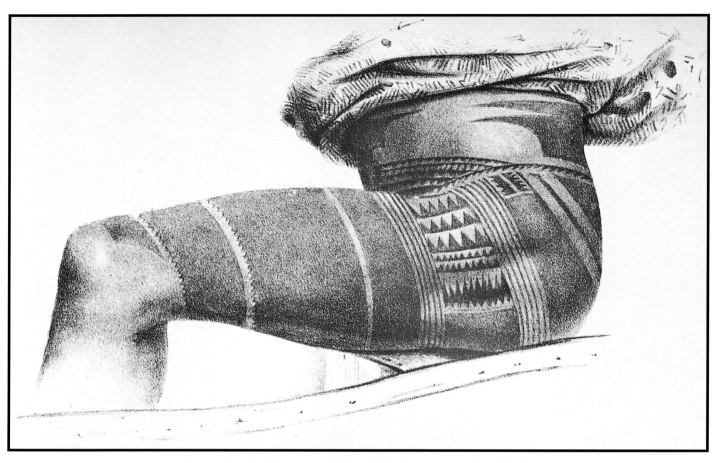

Engraving of a Tongan man's thigh. This picture, drawn from life during Captain Dumont d'Urville's voyage of the *Astrolabe*, is the only visual account left of a traditional Tongan male tattoo. Captain Dumont d'Urville became immortalized later in life for his discovery of the Venus de Milo on Melos.

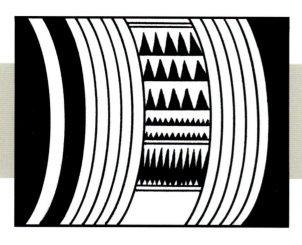

TONGA

Tonga is comprised of 172 islands with a land area of approximately 270 miles, all being historically linked with the same culture and language. Forming three main groups, the island of Tongatapu or "Sacred Tonga" gives part of its name to the entire group, its present-day capital of Nuku'alofa lying to the south. To the north are the islands of Vava'u and in the center the many islands of the Ha'apai, the center of traditional arts and crafts.

The group forms two parallel chains stretching two hundred miles north-northeast/south-southwest of Fiji, with the islands of Samoa south-southwest, Tonga completing the southern apex of this culturally linked triangle. The westerly chain is composed of several volcanic peaks, many being quite active: The island of Tofua, with its large freshwater lake, is in a near-constant state of activity.[1] The rest of the islands in this group are mostly coralline in nature with many in the Ha'apai very low and exposed to the sea.

Due to the proximity to the equator, all of the islands enjoy a warm tropical climate with the average temperature between 70 and 85 degrees Fahrenheit. Like neighboring Samoa and Fiji, hurricanes occasionally occur in the summer months, sometimes with devastating results. The islands receive approximately 70 to 80 inches of rain per year on average, but in the Ha'apai there have been years of severe droughts. The soil on most islands is fertile and intensely cultivated with a wide range of crops grown, with taro, sweet potatoes, bananas and yams being the staples.

Like nearby Fiji and Samoa, ancestors of modern-day Tongans are part of the *Lapita* culture, having migrated from Fiji sometime between 2500 and 300 BC. Little is known of this culture, with dentate-stamped pottery being the only visible archaeological remains found.

In one of the more interesting traditions in Polynesia, prior to the advent of Christianity the Tongans believed that the god Tangaloa[2] climbed down from the sky on a ironwood tree and copulated with a woman of an earlier population who all had descended from a worm. The child from this union, known as *aho'eitu,* half-man and half-god, was to be the first king of Tonga. A celestial half-brother of the king or *Tu'i Tonga* became head of the "second house," accompanied by four ceremonial attendants to the king, known as *falefa,* all of whom were elevated above commoners, providing a rigid basis for Tongan social structure.[3]

Tapu regulations governing high chiefs were complex and strictly enforced. It has been stated, for instance, that if a *Tu'i Tonga* entered a man's house the personal sanctity of the former would make the premises uninhabitable by ordinary mortals.[4] As in the rest of Polynesia, penalties for breaking *tapu* rules were severe, occasionally resulting in death.

At the contact period, Tongans lived in households dispersed among their vast plantations. Houses were wood-framed affairs consisting of one room with leaf thatching and mat walls. Three types were known: the dwelling house *fale nofoanga,* the store house *fale felioko* and the cook house *fale beito.*

Like its nearby neighbors, artistic pursuits were varied with the title of *tufunga* given to the respected craftsmen. Tongan canoe builders were famous for their craftsmanship, resulting in frequent trade with nearby Fiji and Samoa. War clubs and headrests or *kali* were some of the finest produced in Polynesia, employing great skills in workmanship. Fiber and textile arts were ranked equally to that of the carving traditions. Women wove complex baskets or *kato* along with fine pandanus mats. Decorated barkcloth or *ngatu* was also produced, being the equivalent of their artistic counterpart - men's decorated war clubs.

The art of tattoo was mainly limited to men and was applied only to the body between the waist and the thighs. The traditional dress of both sexes was a long kilt or *vala* made of barkcloth or woven pandanus matting. This was wrapped around the waist, falling between the knees. A man of little or no wealth would wear a less elegant loincloth passed between the legs and wrapped around the waist.

The first European to sight the Tongan Islands was the Dutch entrepreneur Jacob Le Maire (1585-1616), who, in 1616 while on a private expedition of his own, sighted the northern islands, the visit being marred by bloodshed.[5] The Dutch explorer Abel Tasman was the next to sight and visit the southern islands of the group in 1643, his encounter being much more peaceful and pleasant. In one of the first encounters with the Tongan people he states:

> With the men came many women aboard; some were uncommonly big, and among them were two fearful giantesses, one of whom had a moustache.

They fell in love with the wound-healer (ships surgeon) and grasped him round the neck, each desiring fleshly intercourse... Some women took off their clothes and bartered items for nails. Others felt the sailors shamelessly in the trouser-front, and indicated that they wished to have intercourse, while the men of the island incited our ship's company to such transgressions.

It was all too much for the puritanical Dutch who left after several weeks with their water-casks full and stores replenished.

The next person to report seeing the islands of Tonga was the Englishman Samuel Wallis, sighting the northern islands in 1767. However, it was the celebrated Captain James Cook who left us with the most detailed accounts of Tonga during his second and third voyages of discovery. Although Cook found the islands peaceful[6] during his visits, the situation changed dramatically when the first missionaries arrived aboard the ship *Duff* in 1799. It was a time of war caused by high-ranking rivalries that continued sporadically for several decades to come. In a fit of desperation, the survivors of the London Missionary Society's expedition were taken off the islands in the following year.

One of the most vivid accounts of this time period comes from William Mariner,[7] who at age 14 went to sea on the privateer *Port au Prince*. While in the Ha'apai group, after several days of friendly trading the ship was taken at Lifuka by 300 Tongans under the leadership of the powerful chief Finau. In the course of the attack and plunder 26 crewmen were killed, with several survivors including the young Mariner being adopted by the Tongans. Under the protection of Finau, Mariner became fluent in the Tongan language and assisted the chief with the use of the cannons from the ship *Port au Prince* against his rivals in Vava'u and Tongatapu. After nearly four years in Tonga he returned to England on the ship *Favourite,* arriving in 1811 after several years of great adventures. Upon his return he was interviewed by a London doctor, John Mariner, with the results being published as one of the great classics of the South Seas, *An Account of the Natives of The Tonga Islands in the South Pacific Ocean.*

After Mariner's visit the islands were not frequently visited due to the well-known hostility of the inhabitants. It was during the time period of the 1820s that Taufa'ahua, a powerful chief, achieved much political and military power. With the arrival of the Wesleyan missionaries in 1828, he chose to adopt their faith, being baptized George Tupou in 1831. Converting as a matter of political convenience, not a matter of faith, the wars continued, bracing the new religion against the old order. With the help of the missionaries he defeated the incumbent *Tu'i Tonga* in 1852 proclaiming himself King of all of Tonga. Living for another 39 years, he was remarkable for the fact he was able to keep Tonga independent of direct annexation from the major maritime powers, this being done with the help and advice of the missionary Shirley Baker.

Treaties of mutual protection were then signed with many of the major powers towards the end of the century, the most important being with Great Britain.[8]

Today the Kingdom of Tonga is the only Pacific Island that has not been colonized by a foreign power, being a member of the British Commonwealth since 1970. Its current monarch, King Tupou IV, can trace his genealogy back to Tangaloa. A remarkable man, he governs his island kingdom with a firm hand, based upon traditional Polynesian values blended with Christianity and modern technology. Under the King's guidance there is still an importance placed on the land, which can never be sold, thus helping keep the deeply rooted Polynesian culture alive for future generations.

Tongan Tattooing – *Ta-tatau*

The little that is known about Tongan tattooing is provided by various accounts left to us by explorers and missionaries. During his second voyage, on the island of Tongatapu in October 1773, Captain James Cook describes tattooing for the first time:

> The same Custom of Tattowing (inlaying the Colour of black in the skin in such a manner as to be indelible) prevails here as the other isles, the men are tattowed from the Middle of the thigh up to above the hips, even their gentiles, I am told do not escape. The Women are not tattowed in this manner, they have it only slitely done on the Arms hands and fingers.

On the third voyage, the account of Cook's surgeon, William Anderson,[9] leaves us with another description of tattooing in Tonga:

> The men are stained from about the middle of the belly to about half way down the thighs with a deep blue colour. This is done by what we might call puncturation or ingraining with a little flat bone instrument cut full of fine teeth & fix'd in a handle. It is dipt into the staining mixture, which is prepard from the soot of the Dooedooe and struck into the skin with a bit of stick untill the blood sometimes follows, and by that means leaves such indelible marks that time cannot efface them. They trace in this manner the various lines & figures that fancy suggests which in some are very elegant either from their variety or disposition, but as the practice is quite universal it does not appear whether it is intended as an ornament, or merely a compliance with one of those old customs for whose institution no satisfactory reason can be given in after times. The women have none of this about their bodys but often a few small lines or spots on the inside of their hands.

It was William Mariner's account that probably is the most accurate:

> The instrument used for the purpose of this operation somewhat resembles a small-tooth comb. They have several kinds, of different degrees of breadth, from six up to fifty or sixty teeth. They are made of bone of the wing of the wild duck. Being

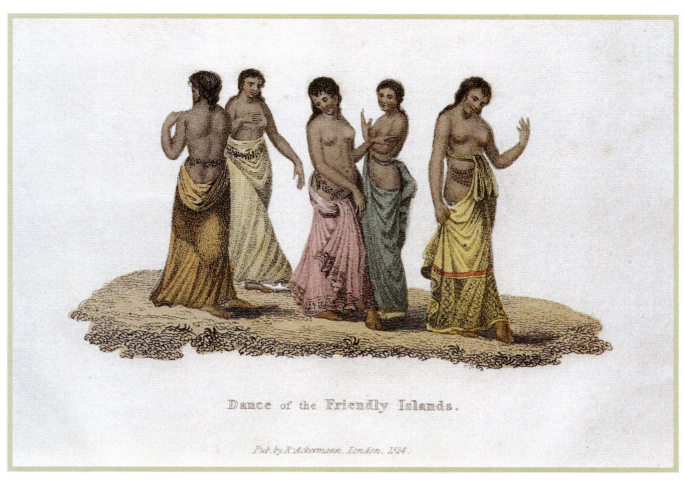

Engraving entitled "Dance of the Friendly Islands." From *The World in Miniature - South Sea Islands*, published in 1824 in London, Frederick Shorbel editor. A rather fanciful depiction of female tattooing and attire.

dipped in a mixture of soot and water, the outline of the tattow is first marked off before the operator begins to puncture, which he afterwards does by strikng the points of the instrument with a small stick cut out of green branch of the cocoa-nut tree. When the skin begins to bleed, which it quickly does, the operator occasionally washes off the blood with cold water, and repeatedly goes over the same places. As this is a very painful process, but a small portion of it is done at once, giving the patient (who may be justly so called) intervals of three or four days rest, so that it is frequently two months before it is completely finished. The parts tattowed are from within two inches of the knees up to about three inches above the umbillicus. There are certain patterns or forms of the tattow, known by district names, and the individual may choose which he likes.

These early narratives provide very little information as to why Tongans actually were tattooed, but like other areas in Polynesia it probably was partially as a protective seal or wrapping. Mariner saw it as a form of clothing during his several years' stay in Tonga, suggesting that Tongan men would feel indecent if they were not tattooed.[10] Tattoo, also a mark of rank, would occasionally signify in its absence a high degree of status as was evident in the case of the *Tu'i Tonga* encountered on Cook's third voyage.

Today most scholars agree that early *Lapita* designs were the basis for tattoo and war club patterns and decoration, with every male of social standing receiving a tattoo before reaching adulthood. As in Samoa, women generally rejected non-tattooed men for being sexually undesirable. The buttocks, thighs and the arches of the loins were tattooed, with the penis and anus the favorite areas of young Tongan males of chiefly rank. These last two areas represent a tremendous indifference to pain, thus increasing the person's status.[11] The tattoo artist or *tufunga ta-tatau* would sometimes apply eccentric forms of tattoo, especially in the case of chiefs, great warriors or priests, all distinguishing them in some special way from the commoners. Like neighboring Fiji, Tongan men painted their bodies for battle, complete with uncolored barkcloth turbans.

Tattooing of women in Tonga was similar to that of Samoa, with the exception being that it was limited to the hands and wrists. Why no other areas of the body were tattooed remains unknown.

The decline of tattoo in Tonga was very rapid; with the arrival of the missionaries, it was expressly forbidden. Samoa, on the other hand, never abandoned the practice. Today tattooing in Tonga is non-existent with no contemporary accounts of it being practiced in over 150 years, providing a mysterious end to a once glorious art form.[12]

Tongan war club. This unusual and rare object is finely carved throughout with both geometric and figural design elements of men and animals, all being intricately incised. Collected by Captain Cook on his third voyage, it became part of his own collection, suggesting it was a gift from the Tu'i Tonga himself. It is shown here to demonstrate the geometric design elements, all being similar to traditional Tongan tattoo patterns. Dr. Adrienne Kaeppler, Curator of Oceanic Art at the Smithsonian Institution, has written extensively about this club in her book *From the Stone Age to the Space Age in Two Hundred Years*, stating, "Its beauty, history, and significance make it one of the most important examples of Tongan art in the world." Height: 43-1/2 inches.

Endnotes

[1] The author is one of the few people ever to land by seaplane in the fresh-water lake of Tofua, hiking to the active summit only to be met with a flurry of volcanic activity. The fresh-water lake is thermally heated, consisting of many hot and cold spots.

[2] *Tangaloa* is the only god of the four major Polynesian deities recognized by the Tongans, revering him as the sky god. In the Vava'u group of islands he is credited with hauling up all of Vava'u from beneath the sea. The common or ordinary people in Tonga were known as *tu'a*, today they are known as *kakai*.

[3] The king or *Tu'i Tonga* was accompanied by ceremonial attendants known as *matapule*. The chiefs were known as *'eiki*.

[4] This according to Irving Goldman in his book entitled *Ancient Polynesian Society*, published in Chicago in 1970.

[5] Le Maire left Holland on June 14, 1615, for the Southern Ocean (as it was called during this time period) on a secret for-profit expedition. The ships were the *Eendracht* and the *Hoorn*, the latter eventually being lost in a fire. Although their stop in Tonga was brief, it twice turned bloody. First they seized a Tongan canoe by force, killing and wounding many. Later, off Niuatoputapu, which they named Traitor's Island, their ship was attacked by stone-throwing warriors; in reply the explorers discharged a cannon loaded with musket-balls and nails killing and wounding many.

[6] Captain James Cook was so well received in Tonga that he gave the group the name "The Friendly Islands," this name being used well into the 19th century. In an odd bit of irony, the Tongans actually had been planning to attack and seize his ships, but due to some unusual circumstances that never transpired, Cook leaving earlier than the Tongans anticipated.

[7] William Mariner was born in London in 1791. In Tonga he was given the name Toki Ukamea or iron adze. Today his exploits in Tonga provide us with an in-depth record of Tongan culture at this time of internal strife and conflict.

[8] The influence of the British monarchy was compatible with many Tongan traditions, hence the present-day parliamentary and justice systems. Its structure of nobles and barons also draws directly from this British system.

[9] William Anderson (1748-1778) was the surgeon's mate on the *Resolution*. While in Tonga in July 1777, the young Anderson recorded this description of tattooing in his journal. He was highly admired by Captain Cook.

[10] Some scholars suggest that tattooing thus would make nakedness more socially desirable.

[11] It was reported that King George I (Tupou I) had the head of his penis or *ule* completely tattooed.

[12] Samoa, like Tonga, is a country of deeply religious values, complete with all the various sects of Christianity present and accounted for. Why the art of tattoo was frowned upon in Tonga and not Samoa is still a mystery.

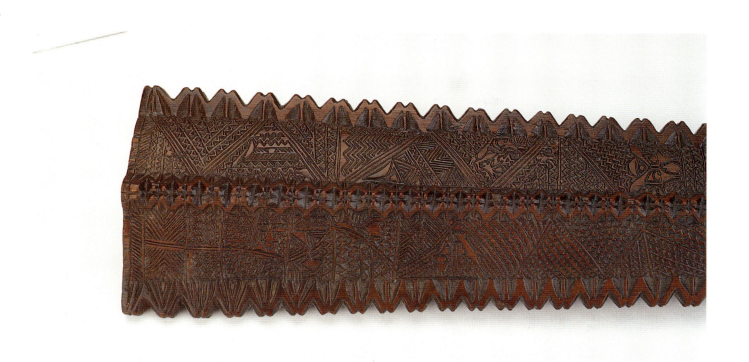
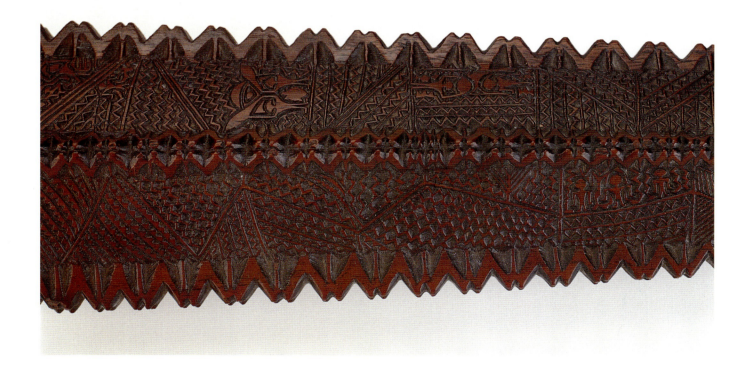
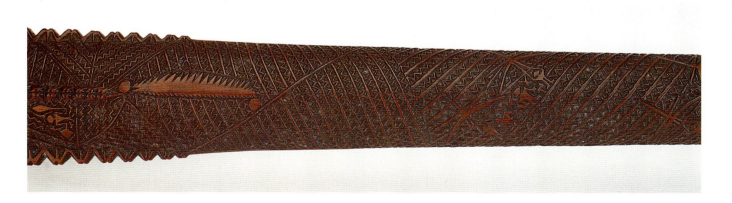

Appendix

Principal Voyages in the Exploration of Polynesia

POLYNESIAN
c. 3500-3000 BC
Purposeful migration from Taiwan/South China coast to Philippines.
c. 3000-2000 BC
Purposeful migration from Philippines to northern coastal New Guinea, Bismarck Archipelago and Solomon Islands.
c. 2000-1200 BC
Purposeful migration from Southern Coastal Melanesia including New Caledonia.
c. 1200-200 BC
Purposeful migration from Melanesia to Fiji, Samoa and Tonga.
c. 200BC-600 AD
Skillful voyaging to Society Islands, Marquesas, Tuamotus, and Cook and Tubuai archipelagos.
c. 600-1000 AD
Purposeful migration to Hawai`i, Easter Island and New Zealand.

SPANISH
16th Century
Magellan 1521- first crossing of the Pacific. Discoveries in the Tuamotus and Micronesia.
Mendana 1595- discovers Marquesas, Santa Cruz and Eastern Caroline Islands.
17th Century
Quiros 1606- discovers Henderson, Ducie and Rakahanga Islands. Additional discoveries in Tuamotus, Banks, New Hebrides, and Gilbert Islands.
18th Century
Bonochea 1772- discoveries in Tuamotus and Austral Islands. Spends time in Society group.

DUTCH
17th Century
Le Maire 1616- discovers seaway to the Pacific south of Cape Horn. Discoveries in Tuamotus, Tonga group, Horne Islands, Bismark Archipelago. Proves insularity of New Guinea.
Tasman 1642- discovers New Zealand and Tasmania. Discoveries in Tuamotus, Tonga group and Ontong Java. Proves Australia does not extend eastward into the Pacific.
18th Century
Roggeveen 1722- discovers Easter Island. Discoveries in Tuamotus and Samoa.

FRENCH
18th Century
Bougainville 1768- discoveries in Tuamotus, Society Islands, New Hebrides and Solomons. His report on the Polynesian way of Tahiti promotes the concept of the Noble Savage.
La Perouse 1787- discoveries in Samoa Group. Discovers Necker Island and French Frigate Shoals north of Hawai`i.

BRITISH
18th Century
Wallis 1767- discoveries in Tuamotus, Society Islands. First landing in Tahiti and Marshall Islands.
Carteret 1767- discovers Pitcarin Island. Discoveries in Tuamotus and Solomons.
Cook 1769- discoveries in Tuamotus, Society Islands and Austral Islands. First circumnavigation of New Zealand. Maps east coast of Australia.
Cook 1773- discoveries in the Cook Islands, New Hebrides, Marquesas and New Caledonia.
Cook 1778- discoveries in Cook, Tonga and Austral Islands. Discovery of Christmas Island and Hawaiian group. Last of Cook's three voyages with his death in Hawai`i.
Bligh 1789- discovers Bounty Islands. Discoveries in Fiji and Banks Island. *Bounty* mutineers discover Raratonga in 1793.
Vancouver 1791- discovers Chatham Islands. Detailed survey of the coast of British Columbia and Alaska.
19th Century
Fitzroy 1831- discoveries in Tuamotus. Charles Darwin's research while aboard this voyage results in book *Origin of Species*.

AMERICAN
18th Century
Ingraham 1791- discoveries in the Marquesas Islands.

RUSSIAN
19th Century
Kotzebue 1815- discoveries in Tuamotus and Marshall Islands. Discovery of Bikini atoll.
Bellinghausen 1820- second circumnavigation of Antarctica. Discoveries in Fiji and Tuamotu Islands.

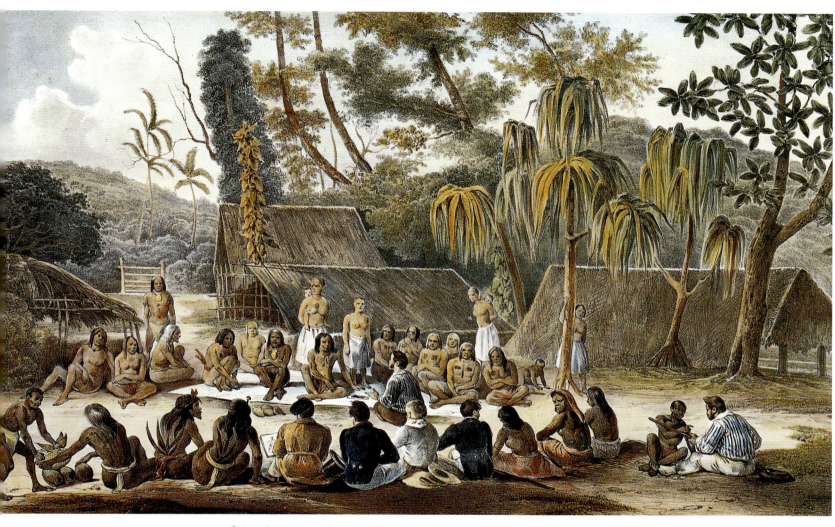

Original engraving from the French voyage of the *Astrolabe*, 1826-1829, Captain Dumont d'Urville commander. This picture shows members of the crew seated before the chiefs of the island of Tikopia, a Polynesian outlier. Tikopians were well known for their wide use of tattoo, which is illustrated in this remarkable image.

Bibliography

Allen, Tricia.
1991 *European Explorers and Marquesan Tattooing: The Wildest Island Style*. Honolulu.

Angas, G.F.
1846 *The New Zealanders Illustrated*, 2 volumes. London.

Arago, Jacques.
1823 *Narrative of a Voyage Round the World*. London
1840 *Souvenirs d' un avengle, voyage autour du monde*. 2 volumes. Paris.

Arredondo B., Ana Maria
1998 *The Art of Tattoo on Rapa Nui*. Proceedings of the Fourth International Conference on Easter Island and East Polynesia. Los Osos.

Balfour, M.C. (ed.)
1903 *From Saranac to the Marquesas and Beyond*. London.

Barrow, Terence
1969 *Maori Wood Sculpture of New Zealand*. Wellington.
1973 *Art and Life in Polynesia*. Tokyo.
1979 *The Art of Tahiti and the Neighbouring Society, Austral, and Cook Islands*. London.
1984 *An Illustrated Guide to Maori Art*. Honolulu.

Beaglehole, J.C. (ed.)
1962/67 *The Journals of Captain James Cook on His Voyages of Discovery*. 5 volumes. Cambridge.

Bellwood, Peter
1978 *The Polynesians: Prehistory of an island people*. London.

Bennett, Frederick
1840 *Narrative of a Whaling Voyage round the globe from the year 1833-1836*. London.

Best, Elsdon
1904 "The Uhi-Maori, or Native Tattooing Instruments." *The Journal of the Polynesian Society*. 13:166-72.
1924 *The Maori*. 2 volumes. Wellington.

Buck, Peter H.
1957 *Arts and Crafts of Hawaii*. Bishop Museum Special Publication #45. Honolulu.

Buzacott, Rev. Aaron
1866 *Mission life in the islands of the Pacific*. London.

Choris, Louis
1822 *Voyage Pittoresque Autour du Monde*. Paris.

Churchill, William
1912 *Easter Island: The Rapanui Speech and the Peopling of Southeast Polynesia*. Washington, D.C.

Cook, James and James King
1784 *A Voyage to the Pacific Ocean... 1776-1780*. London.

Cowan, J.
1921 "Maori Tattooing Survival: Some Notes on Moko." *The Journal of the Polynesian Society*. 30: 241-45.
1930 *Pictures of Old New Zealand: The Partridge Collection Of Maori Paintings by Gottfried Lindauer*. Auckland.

Cruise, R.H.
1824 *Journal of a Ten Month's Residence in New Zealand*. London.

Danielsson, Bengt
1981 *Tahiti Autrefois*. Papeete.

Dening, Greg
1980 *Islands and Beaches: Discourse on a Silent Land - Marquesas*. Honolulu.

Dixon, George A.
1789 *A Voyage Round the World...1785-1788*. London

Dodd, Edward
1967 *Polynesian Art*. London.

Duperrey, L.I.
1826 *Voyage autour du Monde sur la Corvette de sa Majeste La Coquille pendant les Annees 1822, 1823, 1824, et 1825*. Paris.

D'Urville, J.S.C. Dumont
1830/33 *Voyage de la Corvette l'Astrolabe Execute par Ordre du Roi pendant les Annees1826, 1827, 1828, 1829*. 2 volumes. Paris.
1842 *Voyage Pittoresque Autour du monde*. 2 volumes. Paris.

Earl, H.
1832 *A Narrative of a Nine Month's Residence in New Zealand in 1827*. London.

Ehlers, Otto E.
1895 *Samoa, die Perle der Sudsee*. Berlin.

Ellis, William
1783 *An Authentic Narrative of a Voyage performed by Capt. Cook and Capt Clerke*. London.

Ellis, Rev. William
1827 *Narrative of a Tour Through Hawaii*. London.
1831 *Polynesian Researches*. 4 volumes. London.

Emory, Kenneth P.
1946 "Hawaiian Tattooing." *Bishop Museum Occasional Papers* 18 (17). Honolulu.

Erskine, E.E.
1853 *Journal of a Cruise of the Western Pacific*. London.

Ferdon, Edwin N.
1981 *Early Tahiti as the Explorers Saw It 1767-1797*. Tucson.
1993 *Early Observations of Marquesan Culture 1595-1813*. Tucson.

Forment, Francina
1990 *Le Motif de l'oiseau dans la sculpture en bois traditionelle de l'ile de Paques*. Museum of Art and History. Brussels.

Gauguin, Paul
1921 *Lettres De Gauguin a Andre Fontainas*. Paris.
1924 *Noa Noa, Voyage de Tahiti*. Paris.

Geary, C.M. & Webb, Virginia-Lee
1998 *Delivering Views, Distant Cultures in Early Postcards*. Washington, D.C.

Geiseler, Wilhelm (Wm. & G. Ayres Trans.)
1994 *Geiseler's Easter Island Report*. Social Science Research Institute, University of Hawaii. Honolulu.

Gell, Alfred
1993 *Wrapping in Images: Tattooing in Polynesia.* Oxford.

Gill, Rev. William Wyatt
1894 *From darkness to light in Polynesia.* London.

Goldman, Irving
1970 *Ancient Polynesian Society.* Chicago.

Green, Roger C.
1979 "Early Lapita Art from Polynesia and Island Melanesia: Continuities in Ceramic, Barkcloth, and Tattoo Decorations." In Sidney M. Mead (ed.) *Exploring the Visual Arts of Oceania.* Honolulu.

Hambly, W.D.
1925 *The History of Tattooing and its Significance.* London.

Hamilton, A.
1896 *The Art and Workmanship of the Maori Race in New Zealand.* Dunedin.

Handy, W.C.
1921 *Tattooing in the Marquesas.* Bishop Museum Bulletin #1. Honolulu.

Henry, Teuira
1928 *Ancient Tahiti.* Bishop Museum Bulletin #48. Honolulu

Heyerdahl, Thor
1975 *The Art of Easter Island.* Garden City.

Ivory, Carol
1990 *Marquesan Art in the Early Contact Period 1774-1821.* University of Washington Dissertation, 1990.

Kaeppler, Adrienne
1978 *Artificial Curiosities.* Bishop Museum Press. Special Publication #65. Honolulu.
1982 "Genealogy and Disrespect: A Study of Symbolism in Hawaiian Images." *RES* 3:82-107.
1985 "Hawaiian Art and Society: Traditions and Transformations." In *Transformations of Polynesian Culture.* Anthony Hooper and Judith Huntsman (eds.). Auckland.
1997 "Polynesian and Micronesian Art." *Oceanic Art.* 21-158.
1998 *From the Stone Age to the Space Age in Two Hundred Years.* Nuku'alofa.

Lee, Georgia
1992 *The Rock Art of Easter Island.* Los Angeles.

Mackaness, George
1931 *The Life of Vice-Admiral William Bligh.* New York.

Marchand, Etienne Nicholas
1961 "Journal de Bord du capitaine Etienne Marchand." *Bulletin de la Societe des etudes oceaniennes.* 11:247-60.

Marquardt, Carl
1899 *Die Tatowirung in Samoa.* Berlin.

Martin, John
1817 *An Account of the Natives of the Tonga Islands, in the South Pacific Ocean.* London.

Metraux, Alfred
1971 *Ethnology of Easter Island.* Bishop Museum Bulletin #160. Honolulu.

Murray-Oliver, A.
1968 *Augustus Earle in New Zealand.* Christchurch
1969 *Captain Cook's Artists in the Pacific 1769-1799.* Auckland.

King, Michael
1972 *Moko: Maori Tattooing in the 20th Century.* Wellington.

Kotzebue, Otto von
1821 *A Voyage of Discovery into the South Seas and Bearing Straits.* 3 volumes. London.

Kramer, Augustin
1902 *Die Samoa Inselin.* 2 volumes. Stuttgart.
1906 *Hawaii, Ostmikronesien, und Samoa.* Stuttgart.

Malte-Brun, C.
1811 *Sur le tatouage en general et particulierement sur celui des insulaires de Noukahiwa.* Paris.

Nicholas, J.L.
1817 *Narrative of a Voyage to New Zealand performed in the years 1814 and 1815 in company With the Rev. Samuel Marsden, Principal Chaplain of New South Wales.* 2 volumes. London.

O'Brian, Patrick
1987 *Joseph Banks.* London.

Oliver, Douglas
1974 *Ancient Tahitian Society.* 3 volumes. Honolulu.

Orbell, Margaret
1994 *The Illustrated Encyclopedia of Maori Myth and Legend.* Canterbury.

Orliac, Michel & Catherine
1995 *The Silent Gods: Mysteries of Easter Island.* London.
1995 *Bois Sculptes De L'ile De Paques.* Marseille.

Porter, David
1822 *Journal of a Cruise Made to the Pacific Ocean in the United States Frigate Essex, 1812, 1813, 1814.* 2 Volumes. Philadelphia.

Portlock, Nathaniel
1789 *A Voyage Round the World...1785-1788.* London.

Robley, Major-General
1896 *Moko; or Maori Tattooing.* London.

Rose, Roger
1971 *The Material Culture of Ancient Tahiti.* Unpublished thesis. Harvard University. Cambridge, Mass.

Routledge, Mrs. Scoresby
1919 *The Mystery of Easter Island.* London.

Rubin, Arnold (ed.)
1988 *Marks of Civilization.* University of California, Los Angeles.

St. Cartmail, Keith
1997 *The Art of Tonga.* Honolulu.

Saquet, Jean-Louis
1989 *The Tahiti Handbook.* Papeete.

Savage, John
1807 *Some Account of New Zealand.* London.
Simmons, David
1976 *The Great New Zealand Myth: A Study of the Discovery and Origin Traditions of the Maori.* Wellington.
1986 *Ta Moko: The Art Of Maori Tattoo.* Auckland.
Smith, Bernard
1985 *European Vision and the South Pacific.* New Haven.
Smith, S. P.
1910 *Maori Wars of the Nineteenth Century.* Christchurch.
Steinen, Karl von den
1925/28 *Die Marquesaner und ihre Kunst.* 3 volumes. Berlin.
Stolpe, H.
1891 *Evolution in the Ornamental Art of Savage Peoples.* Rochdale.
1899 "Über die Tatowirung der Osterinsulaner." *Friedlander.* Berlin.
Thomson, Dr. A.S.
1859 *The Story of New Zealand.* 2 volumes. London.
Thomson, William J.
1891 *Report on Easter Island.* Washington, D.C.
Turner, George
1861 *Nineteen Years in Polynesia: Missionary Life, Travel, and Researches.* London.
Van Tilburg, Jo Anne
1992 *HMS Topaze on Easter Island.* British Museum Occasional Paper #73. London.
1993 *Easter Island: Archaeology, Ecology, and Culture.* London.
Von Langsdorff, G.H.
1813 *Voyages and Travels in Various Parts of the World During the Years 1803, 1804, 1805, 1806, 1807.* London.
West, Rev. Thomas
1865 *Ten Years in South-Central Polynesia.* London.
White, John
1889 *The Ancient History of the Maori, his Mythology and Traditions.* 2 volumes. London.
Williams, Rev. John
1837 *A Narrative of Missionary Enterprises in the South Sea Islands.* London.
Wright, O.
1955 *The Voyage of the Astrolabe in 1840.* Wellington.

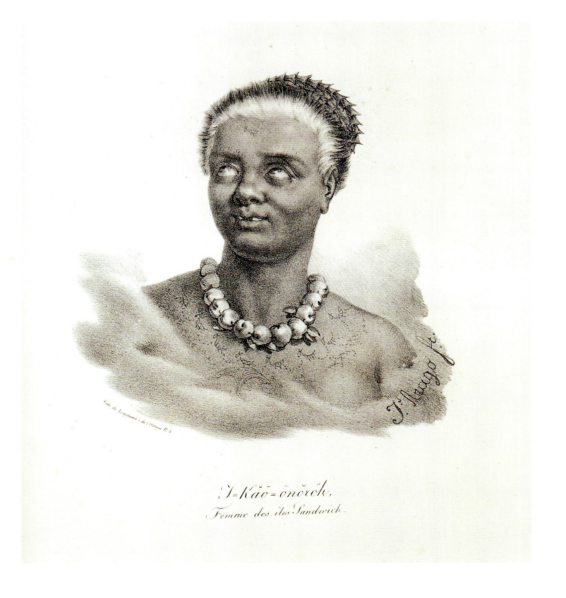

Index

American Board of Commissions for Foreign
    Missions, 88
Anaru Makiwhara, 15
Andrew, Thomas, 176, 191
Arago, Jacques, 86, 89, 91-105
Arioi society, 109, 111, 113
Aterea, 15
Austral Islands, 109, 112, 161
Banks, Sir Joseph, 9, 111, 113, 114
Baptismal tattoo, 15, 27, 47, 85
Bayard Dominick Expedition, 122, 133
Bennett, Frederick, 112, 113
Birdman, 157, 158, 161, 168, 169
Bligh, Captain William, 110, 113
Bougainville, Captain Louis Antoine de, 110, 113, 173
Buck, Sir Peter, 12
Buttock tattoo, 11, 15, 33
Cabri, John Baptiste, 119, 121, 144, 150
Choris, Louis, 106, 162
Church Missionary Society, 47
Colenso, Rev., 76
Cook, Captain James, 7, 9, 12, 15, 30, 43, 49,
    87-90, 107, 108, 110, 111, 113, 115, 118,
    145, 159, 161, 162, 194
d'Urville, Admiral Dumont, 115, 124, 192, 199
Darning needles, 15, 16, 71, 80, 82
Davis, John, 176
Diderot, Denis, 113
Duperrey, Captain Louis Isidore, 44
Dupetit-Thouar, Admiral, 119
Ellis, William, 89, 92, 111
Flaherty, Frances Hubbard, 5, 179
Forster, 118, 161
Gauguin, Paul, 111, 119
Gauthier, Lucien, 141
Geiseler, Captain Wilhelm, 161, 162
Goldie, Charles F., 36, 37, 50, 62, 85
Gonzalez, Felipe, 159
Guide, Eileen and Georgina, 82, 83
Hawaiki, 9
Herewini, 15
Heyerdahl, Thor, 161
Hinemoa, 35
Hingi Hika, 11
Hoare, Mrs. S., 148
Hodges, William, 145
Homes, Frank, 120, 124, 140
Hori Ngakapa, 39
Hotu Matua, 157
Ka'ioi, 144
Kahukuhu, 15, 72
Kahunas, 87, 88
Kamareira Te Hau Takiri Wharepapa, 40
Kamehameha I, 88, 93, 98
Kapikapi, 36

Kapu, 88, 90
King Tupou IV, 194
Kohere, 11
Kohimarama conference, 24
Koru, 13, 33
Kramer, Dr. Augustin Friedrich, 104, 191
Krusenstern, 118
Lapita, 7, *173, 193*
Le Perouse, 159
Lindauer, Gottfried, 67, 21
London Missionary Society, 111, 173, 178
Loti, Pierre, 163
Mahuta Te Teko, 50, 74
Malietoa Vaiinupo, 173
Mana, 9, 31, 40, 88, 116, 119, 130, 158, 175
Maori Wars, 11, 15, 16, 25, 28, 62, 64
Marchand, Captain E., 118
Mariner, William, 194, 195
Marquardt, Carl, 177, 180-190
Mead, Margaret, 173, 178
Mellville, Herman, 119, 122
Mendana, 117, 123
Mere Werohia, 37
Merrett, Joseph Jenner, 33
Metraux, 161, 162
Moai kava kava, 157, 160, 169
Moai tagnata, 169, 170, 171
Moai, 158, 160, 161
Moana of the South Seas, 5
Mohi a Te Ngu, 74
Musket trade, 11, 13, 16, 18, 30
Navigator Islands, 173, 178
Noble Savage, 110, 113
Omai, 30, 108, 110, 117, 205
Orongo, 158, 160, 161
Pai Marire, 31
Parkinson, Syndey, 15, 49
Patuone, 43
Penny-*haka*, 48
Petroglyph, 95, 161
Porter, Captain David, 127, 144
Pou tokomanawa, 16, 34, 35
Preserved heads, 11, 17, 18
Puhoro, 15
Pukaki, 32
Rangatira, 9
Robarts, Edward, 119
Robley, Major General Horatio Gordon, 17, 28,
    29, 34, 68
Roggeveen, Jacob, 158, 162, 173
Rongorongo tablets, 7
Rousseau, Jean-Jacques, 113
Samwell, David, 90
Savage, John, 53
Spitz, Charles, 132

Stevenson, Robert Louis, 122, 174
Stilt step, 126
Stolpe, Hjalmar, 166
Stuart, Samuel, 43
Tame Poata, 15
Tapu, 9, 11, 13, 119, 158, 173
Taraia Ngakuti Te Tumuhuia, 61
Tasman, Abel, 9, 193
Taupou, 173, 179
Taurau Kukupa, 41
Tawhiao Potatau Wherowhero, 41, 65, 85
Taylor, Reverend Richard, 13, 15
Te Akau, 75
Te Kooti, 76
Te Pehi Kupe, 15, 30
Te Rangikaheke, 12
Te Rau, Kereopa, 31
Te Tuhi, 85
The Great Omi, 205

Thomson, William, 161, 164
Thomson, A.S., 15
Tiki, 119, 126
Tohunga, 11
Treaty of Waitangi, 11, 15, 119
Tree fern, 13, 74
Tu'i Tonga, 193-195
Turner, Reverend George, 178
Tutanekai, 45
Tutua, 9
U.S. Exploring Expedition, 92
U'u, 118, 124, 126
Volkner, C.S., 31, 34
Von Langsdorff, G.H., 117, 120, 130, 142, 153-155
Waitara, 11, 15
Wallis, Samuel, 110, 194
Webber, John, 107
Whakairo tattoo, 15
Williams, Reverend John, 114

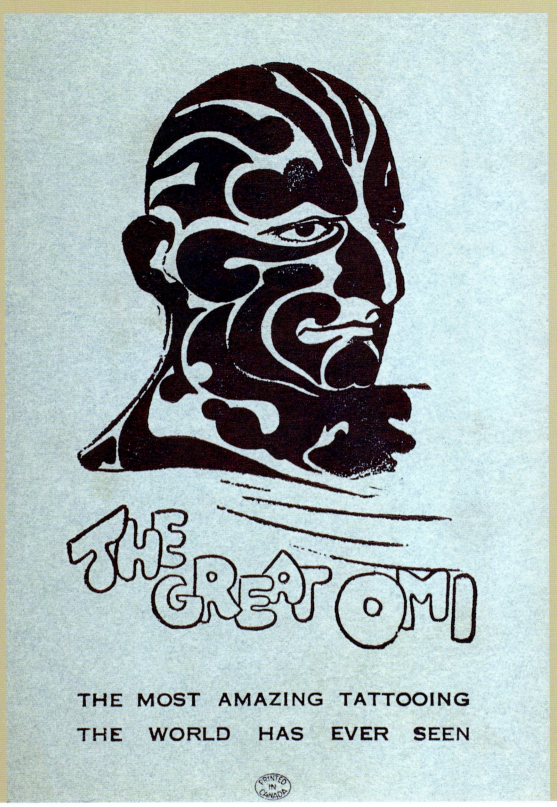

Original postcard of The Great Omi, whose real name was Major Horace Ridler, one of the most famous circus tattoo attractions of all time. He toured throughout Europe in the 1920s, then moved to the United States where he joined Ripley's "Believe It Or Not Show" in 1938. He also worked for Ringling Brothers' Barnum and Bailey Circus where he was one of the highest paid performers. Born into a wealthy British family, he was well educated, joined the Army, and was decorated for heroism in the First World War. After an honorable discharge, he drifted around for many years and realized the only occupation that appealed to him was the circus. Lacking any skills appropriate to the job, he contacted London's most famous tattooist, George Burchett, who agreed to apply a zebra-like pattern of stripes over his entire body; the process took over a year at three sessions a week. The Great Omi died in 1969 at the age of 77.

This image is included to show that there may be a "popular culture" connection that influenced the Major to adopt a stage name similar to that of Omai, of Captian Cook's voyages fame, who was the first tattooed Polynesian to set foot in England in the 18th century.

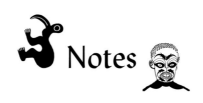
Notes